Dirk Lanzerath, Marcella Rietschel (eds.)
Ethics of Research Involving Minors

MEDIZIN-ETHIK
MEDICAL ETHICS

Schriftenreihe des Arbeitskreises
Medizinischer Ethik-Kommissionen
in der Bundesrepublik Deutschland e. V.

herausgegeben von

Dirk Lanzerath

in Verbindung mit

Joerg Hasford
und
Sebastian Graf von Kielmansegg

Band 29

Ethics of Research Involving Minors
A European Perspective

edited by

Dirk Lanzerath and Marcella Rietschel

LIT

Cover Image:
Bildnummer: 7353
Künstler: Macke, August, 1887–1914
Bildtitel: Kinder im Garten. 1912.
Maße: 89,2 × 71,1 cm
Standort: Bonn, Städtisches Kunstmuseum
Foto: © Reni Hansen – ARTOTHEK

The present volume received funding from the European Community's Seventh Framework Programme (FP7/2007–2013) under grant agreement no. 602450 (IMAGEMEND).

This book is printed on acid-free paper.

Bibliographic information published by the Deutsche Nationalbibliothek
The Deutsche Nationalbibliothek lists this publication in the Deutsche Nationalbibliografie; detailed bibliographic data are available on the Internet at http://dnb.d-nb.de.

ISBN 978-3-643-90975-6 (pb)
ISBN 978-3-643-95975-1 (PDF)

© **LIT VERLAG** Dr. W. Hopf Berlin 2018
Verlagskontakt:
Fresnostr. 2 D-48159 Münster
Tel. +49 (0) 2 51-62 03 20
E-Mail: lit@lit-verlag.de   http://www.lit-verlag.de

Auslieferung:
Deutschland: LIT Verlag, Fresnostr. 2, D-48159 Münster
Tel. +49 (0) 2 51-620 32 22, E-Mail: vertrieb@lit-verlag.de
E-Books sind erhältlich unter www.litwebshop.de

Contents

Preface 1
Dirk LANZERATH and Marcella RIETSCHEL

Ethical, Legal, and Social Implications of Psychiatric Genetic
Research: Examples of Challenges Encountered within the
Psychiatric Imaging Genetics Project IMAGEMEND 5
Marcella RIETSCHEL, Jana STROHMAIER, Noemi LEMME,
Stephanie WITT

Use of Population-based Samples in Psychiatric Genetics: Ethical
Considerations 33
Christina M. HULTMAN, Viktoria JOHANSSON

Ethics and the Research with Minors – A European Perspective:
Challenges of Pediatric Clinical Research 39
Pirkko LEPOLA

Protection of Minors in Research under the new European Union
Regulations 65
Scarlett JANSEN

Ethical Issues on Research with Minors and Challenges for
Research Ethics Committees 77
Dirk LANZERATH

KIDS Barcelona: Young Persons' Advisory Group Focused in
Clinical Research and Innovation Projects 91
Begonya Nafria ESCALERA, Joana Claverol TORRES

The Ethical Principles Underpinning the Participation of Young
People in the Development of Paediatric Clinical Research 101
Jennifer PRESTON, Pamela DICKS, Begonya Nafria ESCALERA,
Segolene GAILLARD

Young People, Deliberation, and Research Ethics: A Film Project
by the Nuffield Council on Bioethics 107
Kate HARVEY

Preface

Dirk LANZERATH and Marcella RIETSCHEL

Research involving minors, i.e. children and adolescents, is an area of controversy within medical ethics and medical law. Minors represent a vulnerable group, for whom particular protective measures are required and who should be excluded from research that does not offer the prospect of direct benefit. However, the exclusion of minors from research into disorders of relevance to their age group precludes the potential for beneficial medical advances. Furthermore, effective prevention strategies for common medical conditions with an origin in childhood and adolescence, such as mental disorders, require the delineation of those who are at increased risk. Therefore, the particular challenge for research ethics committees is to promote, rather than prevent, such research, while ensuring the required level of ethical protection for these vulnerable subjects. This requirement leads to recurring tensions between ethics committees and patient representatives and paediatric researchers, since in some instances these stakeholders consider the decisions of ethics committees overprotective. This dilemma is not restricted to the possible harm caused by clinical interventions, but is also observed in research in other disciplines, including the humanities. In areas such as trauma research, even the completion of questionnaires may have unwanted side-effects. Besides the potential harm conferred through direct study interventions, several important ethical considerations must be addressed when performing research in minors, in particular those surrounding the issue of data protection. In storing the personal data of minors, researchers cannot guarantee the exclusion of later disadvantageous effects. From both an ethical and a legal perspective, non-medical research fields are subject to inadequate regulation compared to the situation existing in clinical research.

When involving minors in research, scientists face the challenge of interpreting and applying fundamental ethical and legal principles within the rapidly changing real-world research setting. The basic ethical and legal issues of research involving minors were addressed in volume 22 of this series. The central foci of the present volume are practical experiences of research involving minors, issues surrounding psychiatric research including adolescents, and the impact of the new European regulations on research involving children and adolescents. In contrast to the situation for adults who are unable to provide consent, the 2014 EU Regulation on Clinical Trials contains no exemption clause for minors. Consequently, member states are not permitted to impose more stringent national regulations that preclude research with group benefits for this age-group. The exemption clause for adults who are unable to provide consent was added as a compromise during the development phase of the 2014 Regulation. Minors were not considered during these discussions, as a group benefit clause for minors had already been included in EU legislation passed in 2001 (Directive 2001/20/EC).

The first chapter of the present volume addresses the practical ethical demands of the IMAGEMEND project. The overarching aims of this EU funded reasearch project, which involves minors, are to improve knowledge of the aetiology om mental illness and clinical management through the discovery of neuroimaging-based diagnostic-, trans-diagnostic-, and predictive markers; and to facilitate the translation of these markers into clinical diagnostics and therapeutics. The IMAGEMEND consortium has collected extensive data on neuroimaging, genetics, environmental risk factors, and clinical phenotypes, and has used these to establish Europe's largest integrated medical research database. In this chapter, *Marcella Rietschel, Jana Strohmaier, Noemi Lemme,* and *Stephanie Witt* describe how psychiatric genetic- and neuroscientific research, which may include adolescent participants, have proven challenging to scientists and ethicists alike. When applying genetic approaches from research into somatic disorders, psychiatric genetic researchers must be aware of the existence of alternative disease concepts and viewpoints – in particular among study participants – since mental illness and somatic disease may be perceived as two very different concepts. A key into mental disorders is that normality is a vital social asset. Deviation from normality on the basis of a psychiatric genetic test result may therefore give rise to stigmatisation.

In the chapter "Use of population-based samples in psychiatric genetics: Ethical considerations", *Christina M. Hultman* and *Viktoria Johansson* consider the findings of a population-based study from Sweden, which emphasise the normative implications of psychiatric genetic research. This empirical investigation explored the attitudes of psychiatric patients towards psychiatric genetic research. The study showed that patients strongly supported schizophrenia research, and had a positive perception of research in general, at that. Psychiatrists typically underestimated the degree of enthuisasm felt by their patients towards research. The study also showed that psychiatrists underestimated the degree to which patients trusted the researcher team, and that patients preferred to make their own judgement of the study protocol when deciding whether to participate. These findings emphasise the importance of autonomy to research patients and suggest: In determining whether a psychiatric patient should participate in a genetic or neuroscientific research project, the opinion of the treating physician, relative, other carer, or societal representative must be balanced against that of the patient.

In the chapter "Ethics and the Research with Minors - A European Perspective", *Pirkko Lepola* presents a paediatric clinical research perspective. She describes the work being conducted by the European Network of Paediatric Research at the European Medicines Agency (Enpr-EMA) to identify solutions to emergent needs and challenges in relation to paediatric clinical trials and the development of medicines for children. The overarching aim of this work is to facilitate communication between paediatric clinical trial stakeholders. This is being achieved by gathering examples of good practice, and developing pragmatic proposals for future directions.

The chapter "Protection of Minors in Research under the new European Union Regulations" by *Scarlett Jansen* is an analysis of the manner in which minors are protected under the new EU regulations, and of the options available to researchers. In particular, the regulations stress that in order to include minors, a clinical trial must either research a treatment for a medical condition that is restricted to minors only, or be essential in terms of confirming data relating to minors. This serves to counteract the unjustified inclusion of minors in clinical research. In conjunction with other protection mechanisms, the regulations are thus intended to ensure that minors can be involved in research without compromising their level of protection.

In the chapter "Ethical Issues on Research with Minors and Challenges for Research Ethics Committees", *Dirk Lanzerath* emphasises that in the research context, ethical standards reflect the attitudes, beliefs, and habits of the respective researchers, which are in turn based on reliable social norms. The ethics framework thus provides a trustworthy research context within a complex social environment. However, when performing research in minors - in contrast to research with adults - the actors must consider the whole system in which the child or adolescent is involved, i.e. family, institutions, and society as a whole. In this respect, research ethics committees act as an important intermediary between science and society, and between the systems of law and politics.

In the chapters "KIDS Barcelona: Young Persons' Advisory Group Focused in Clinical Research and Innovation Projects" and "The Ethical Principles Underpinning the Participation of Young People in the Development of Paediatric Clinical Research", a series of contributors explore the challenges associated with involving young people in the design and development of the clinical research process, and how these challenges can be overcome within the "Young Person's Advisory Group" context. When considering the issue of beneficence in research involving minors, researchers and research ethics committee members should not refer exclusively to theoretical considerations. Experience in Europe suggests that in addition to patient representatives and experienced paediatricians, researchers and research ethics committees should obtain insight and guidance through consultation with minors. In their contribution, *Begonya Nafria Escalera* and *Joana Claverol Torres* report on their practical experience within the Spanish project "KIDS Barcelona", and the demands involved in realising its potential. This project was established within the framework of the European youth advisory groups for clinical research and innovation projects network. *Jennifer Preston, Pamela Dicks, Begonya Nafria Escalera,* and *Segolene Gaillard* highlight the importance of involving young people in the design and development of paediatric clinical research. The authors define young people as individuals between the ages of eleven and eighteen years, who have a history of a medical condition that requires medication, or those who have no current illness, but who are able to represent the more general views and perspectives of young people.

In the chapter "Young People, Deliberation, and Research Ethics: A Film Project by the Nuffield Council on Bioethics", *Kate Harvey* focuses on the 2015 report of the Nuffield Council on Bioethics on ethical issues associated with the involvement of children and young people in clinical research. To inform the report's conclusions, a range of activities with young people were undertaken during the course of a two-year project. These activities included the establishment of a stakeholder group of young people to advise the project team; the devising of an animated film with the guidance of young people; and consultation with young people during the preparation of drafts of the written report and accompanying materials. In addition to these activities, a film initiative compared the responses of young people and adults to ethical issues raised by a fictional research protocol. The chapter describes the film project's aims, methods, and conclusions.

We acknowledge with due appreciation the editorial support provided by Leonie Overwien and Dorothee Güth, and we are also grateful to Christine Schmäl for language revisions and for comments on the text.

The present volume received funding from the European Community's Seventh Framework Programme (FP7/2007-2013) under grant agreement no. 602450 (IMAGEMEND).

Ethical, Legal, and Social Implications of Psychiatric Genetic Research: Examples of Challenges Encountered within the Psychiatric Imaging Genetics Project IMAGEMEND

Marcella RIETSCHEL, Jana STROHMAIER, Noemi LEMME, Stephanie WITT

Challenges of Research into the Biological Causes of Mental Disorders

Mental disorders are common, and often display a chronic relapsing course. In many cases, onset occurs during early adulthood. Mental disorders impose a major burden on affected individuals, relatives and friends, and society in general. At the time of writing, few data are available concerning the underlying pathophysiology of mental illness, and no biological markers are available to guide diagnosis or predict response to medication or outcome. Major national and international scientific endeavours are underway to improve knowledge in this area, and thus facilitate treatment and prevention. As explained below, successful research will require extensive, multidisciplinary collaborations.

The challenges faced by mental health researchers are daunting. Beyond organisational and technical issues, these mainly relate to the ambitious aims of this research field, which are no less than the identification of the genetic/biological factors that underlie mental illness and mental health. Knowledge of these factors may have unforeseen – positive as well as adverse – implications for research participants, patients, persons at risk, and/or society in general. This raises the question of how the potential negative outcomes of such research can be foreseen and minimised.

The Ethical, Legal and Social Implications (ELSI) Research Program was established in 1990 as an integral part of the Human Genome Project (HGP) to foster basic and applied research on the ethical, legal and social implications of genetic and genomic research for individuals, families and communities. ELSI research has addressed many of the issues such as privacy, autonomy, ramification for families, psychosocial impact, discrimination in employment and insurance that must be taken into account when conducting research of this nature. However, science is now progressing at an unprecedented pace. As a result, researchers face a continuous flow of new problems, as well as novel insights into seemingly previously solved problems that must also be addressed. Ultimately, consideration of these issues may lead to new recommendations, guidelines, and legislation. In the meantime, however, while acquiring data for future use, researchers must act in accordance with existing regulations, while attempting to foresee and consider new issues evoked by their research.

Most of the ELSI encountered within research into mental disorders are not unique. Instead, most are also encountered in projects designed to identify diagnostic and predictive markers for complex somatic disorders, such as cancer, diabetes, and cardiovascular disease. However, research into mental disorders carries additional ELSI compared to those encountered in research into somatic disorders: Despite evidence for a substantial genetic component – and one that is in some cases greater than that reported for the aforementioned somatic diseases – mental illnesses such as schizophrenia, bipolar disorder, and attention deficit hyperactivity disorder (ADHD), are not considered somatic disorders within the wider medical community. Discussion of "the myth of mental illness"[1], and of the many controversies surrounding the methodological, epistemological, and even ontological aspects of psychiatric classification and therapy, is beyond the scope of the present article (for insights into this topic, the interested reader is referred to The Philosophy of Psychiatry and Biologism[2]). Therefore, when investigating the genetic and biological aetiology of mental illness, with the same genetic approaches used for research into somatic disorders, researchers must be aware of the existence of controversial viewpoints and disease concepts, in particular those adhered to by study participants.

A further highly relevant ELSI of genetic research into mental disorders is the potential for stigmatisation. The status of normality is a vital social asset (e.g. as a condition of majority, or requirement for social acceptance), and deviation from normality may be associated with stigma. Psychiatric stigma has many facets.[3] As UK psychiatrist Peter Byrne has stated: "to be marked as 'mentally ill' carries internal (secrecy, lower self-esteem and shame) and external (social exclusion, prejudice and discrimination) consequences, all of which are written about under the 'stigma' heading".[4] Within a research project designed to identify diagnostic and predictive markers of mental illness, the potential for stigma (e.g. for individuals identified as carrying, or having transmitted, an increased genetic risk) cannot be ignored. The issue of stigma adds an additional dimension to important ELSI such as the right to privacy and autonomy, particularly when the research involves

---

[1] Szasz, T. S. (1960): *The Myth of Mental Illness*, in: American Psychologist, 15, 113 – 118.
[2] Stier, M., Schoene-Seifert, B., Rüther, M., Muders, S. (2014): *The philosophy of psychiatry and biologism*, in: Frontiers in Psychology 5, 1032.
[3] Gray, A. J. (2002): *Stigma in psychiatry*, in: Jounal of the Royal Society of Medicine 95, 72–76.
[4] Byrne, P. (2001): *Psychiatric Stigma*, in: The British Journal of Psychiatry 178,281–284.

persons who are likely to be especially vulnerable and/or who lack the capacity to provide informed consent, as it is the case in some psychiatric patients or adolescents. To illustrate efforts to address ELSI in research practice, examples from the Psychiatric Imaging Genetics Project IMAGEMEND (IMAging GEnetics for MENtal Disorders) will be presented below.

State-of-the-Art for Research into the Aetiology of Mental Disorders

Search for Genetic Factors

As mentioned above, current knowledge of the pathophysiology of psychiatric disorders is limited. In contrast to most other complex disorders, no objective measure or biological marker – comparable to staging in cancer, blood pressure monitoring in hypertension, or glucose measurement in diabetes – is yet available to assist the diagnostic process or predict the course of the disorder and disease risk. On the other hand, it is well known that genetic factors play a substantial role in the aetiology and course of mental disorders. A long established finding of formal genetic studies is that genetic factors contribute around 80% to the phenotypic variance observed in schizophrenia, bipolar disorder, and ADHD, and around 40% to that observed in major depression and substance use disorders. Researchers therefore consider that the identification of these factors on a molecular genetic level may generate insights into the underlying pathomechanisms, and ultimately facilitate causal interventions and prevention strategies. Nonetheless, this approach has proven less straightforward than anticipated. First, studies of this nature require many more patients than initially envisaged. Genome-wide association studies (GWAS) which use hundred thousands to millions of common genetic variants to identify associations between single-nucleotide polymorphisms (SNPs) and psychiatric disorders, have so far identified a total of only a few hundred genetic risk variants for all psychiatric disorders together. This required the investigation of tens of thousands of patients, and research suggests that many thousands of variants still await detection. Second, research has shown that single-nucleotide variants with large risk effects exist but they are rare. Their detection will require the performance of a more in depth genome-wide search as GWAS do, i.e. genome-wide sequencing, in even larger cohorts than those used hitherto.

Most of the genetic risk variants identified in psychiatric genetic research to date are SNPs, which have a high frequency in the general population, and each single nucleotide polymorphism is associated with only a marginal increase in disease risk. These common risk variants act both in combination with each other, and in conjunction with environmental factors.

Most of the rare variants identified in psychiatric genetic research to date have been in schizophrenia and these are so called copy number variants (CNVs), i.e. genomic duplications or deletions. Here the variation does not affect a single nucleotide but CNVs span hundreds to millions of base-pairs. However, those CNVs found to be associated with schizophrenia, are not schizophrenia-specific, as they also increase the risk for other neurodevelopmental disorders, such as intellectual disability.[5] Although these CNVs have been found at a significantly higher fre-

---

[5] Malhotra, D., Sebat, J. (2012): *CNVs: harbingers of a rare variant revolution in psychiatric genetics*, in: Cell 148, 1223–1241; Marshall, C. R., Howrigan, D. P., Merico, D., Thiruvahindrapuram, B., Wu, W., Greer, D. S., Antaki, D., Shetty, A., Holmans, P. A., Pinto, D., Gujral, M., Brandler, W. M., Malhotra, D., Wang, Z., Fajarado, K. V. F., Maile, M. S., Ripke, S., Agartz, I., Albus, M., Alexander, M., Amin, F., Atkins, J., Bacanu, S. A., Belliveau, R. A., Jr., Bergen, S. E., Bertalan, M., Bevilacqua, E., Bigdeli, T. B., Black, D. W., Bruggeman, R., Buccola, N. G., Buckner, R. L., Bulik-Sullivan, B., Byerley, W., Cahn, W., Cai, G., Cairns, M. J., Campion, D., Cantor, R. M., Carr, V. J., Carrera, N., Catts, S. V., Chambert, K. D., Cheng, W., Cloninger, C. R., Cohen, D., Cormican, P., Craddock, N., Crespo-Facorro, B., Crowley, J. J., Curtis, D., Davidson, M., Davis, K. L., Degenhardt, F., Del Favero, J., DeLisi, L. E., Dikeos, D., Dinan, T., Djurovic, S., Donohoe, G., Drapeau, E., Duan, J., Dudbridge, F., Eichhammer, P., Eriksson, J., Escott-Price, V., Essioux, L., Fanous, A. H., Farh, K. H., Farrell, M. S., Frank, J., Franke, L., Freedman, R., Freimer, N. B., Friedman, J. I., Forstner, A. J., Fromer, M., Genovese, G., Georgieva, L., Gershon, E. S., Giegling, I., Giusti-Rodriguez, P., Godard, S., Goldstein, J. I., Gratten, J., de Haan, L., Hamshere, M. L., Hansen, M., Hansen, T., Haroutunian, V., Hartmann, A. M., Henskens, F. A., Herms, S., Hirschhorn, J. N., Hoffmann, P., Hofman, A., Huang, H., Ikeda, M., Joa, I., Kahler, A. K., Kahn, R. S., Kalaydjieva, L., Karjalainen, J., Kavanagh, D., Keller, M. C., Kelly, B. J., Kennedy, J. L., Kim, Y., Knowles, J. A., Konte, B., Laurent, C., Lee, P., Lee, S. H., Legge, S. E., Lerer, B., Levy, D. L., Liang, K. Y., Lieberman, J., Lonnqvist, J., Loughland, C. M., Magnusson, P. K. E., Maher, B. S., Maier, W., Mallet, J., Mattheisen, M., Mattingsdal, M., McCarley, R. W., McDonald, C., McIntosh, A. M., Meier, S., Meijer, C. J., Melle, I., Mesholam-Gately, R. I., Metspalu, A., Michie, P. T., Milani, L., Milanova, V., Mokrab, Y., Morris, D. W., Muller-Myhsok, B., Murphy, K. C., Murray, R. M., Myin-Germeys, I., Nenadic, I., Nertney, D. A., Nestadt, G., Nicodemus, K. K., Nisenbaum, L., Nordin, A., O'Callaghan, E., O'Dushlaine, C., Oh, S. Y., Olincy, A., Olsen, L., O'Neill, F. A., Van Os, J., Pantelis, C., Papadimitriou, G. N., Parkhomenko, E., Pato, M. T., Paunio, T., Psychosis Endophenotypes International, C., Perkins, D. O., Pers, T. H., Pietilainen, O., Pimm, J., Pocklington, A. J., Powell, J., Price, A., Pulver, A. E., Purcell, S. M., Quested, D., Rasmussen, H. B., Reichenberg, A., Reimers, M. A., Richards, A. L., Roffman, J. L., Roussos, P., Ruderfer, D. M., Salomaa, V., Sanders, A. R., Savitz, A., Schall, U., Schulze, T. G., Schwab, S. G., Scolnick, E. M., Scott, R. J., Seidman, L. J., Shi, J., Silverman, J. M., Smoller, J. W., Soderman, E., Spencer, C. C. A., Stahl, E. A., Strengman, E., Strohmaier, J., Stroup, T. S., Suvisaari, J., Svrakic, D. M., Szatkiewicz, J. P., Thirumalai, S., Tooney, P. A., Veijola, J., Visscher, P. M., Waddington, J., Walsh, D., Webb, B. T., Weiser, M., Wildenauer, D. B., Williams, N. M., Williams, S., Witt, S. H., Wolen, A. R., Wormley, B. K., Wray, N. R., Wu, J. Q., Zai, C. C., Adolfsson, R., Andreassen, O. A., Blackwood, D. H. R., Bramon, E., Buxbaum, J. D., Cichon, S., Collier, D. A., Corvin, A., Daly, M. J., Darvasi, A., Domenici, E., Esko, T., Gejman, P. V., Gill, M., Gurling, H., Hultman, C. M., Iwata, N., Jablensky, A. V., Jonsson, E. G., Kendler, K. S., Kirov, G., Knight, J., Levinson, D. F., Li, Q. S., McCarroll, S. A., McQuillin, A., Moran, J. L., Mowry, B. J., Nothen, M. M., Ophoff, R. A., Owen, M. J., Palotie, A., Pato, C. N., Petryshen, T. L., Posthuma, D., Rietschel, M., Riley, B.

quency in patients with schizophrenia than in the general population, the precise contribution of the identified CNVs to schizophrenia and other psychiatric disorders remains unknown and can only be estimated. Furthermore, these estimates are context dependent. For example, if all affected members of a large multiplex family with schizophrenia carry a hitherto unknown large CNV, while all unaffected members do not, carrier status of this specific CNV in an adolescent member of this family who begins to display non-specific clinical symptoms, such as apathy and depressed mood, has different implications from a psychiatric genetic research perspective than it would in an individual with the same symptoms but no family history, or in a healthy person from the general population (e.g. as detected during a genetic case-control research study).

As outlined above, to date only a very small fraction of the variants that contribute to mental illness have been identified. However, this number is growing steadily due to increasing sample sizes. Investigations into the function of these variants will increase knowledge concerning disease aetiology. So far the majority of the identified variants do not serve as biomarkers of risk, as the contribution of each individual variant to disease risk is small. However, the contribution to disease risk of their combined effects is substantially higher. Panels of genetic markers, such as polygenic risk scores, summarise the combined genetic effect of multiple variants.[6] For example, studies of schizophrenia have shown that individuals with very high polygenic risk scores have a 20% increase in disease risk compared to individuals with very low scores.[7] With the prospect of more risk variants being detected in the future, researchers envisage that the power of prediction will increase, particularly when further disease predictors, such as fam-

---

P., Rujescu, D., Sklar, P., St Clair, D., Walters, J. T. R., Werge, T., Sullivan, P. F., O'Donovan, M. C., Scherer, S. W., Neale, B. M., Sebat, J., Cnv, Schizophrenia Working Groups of the Psychiatric Genomics, C. (2017): *Contribution of copy number variants to schizophrenia from a genome-wide study of 41,321 subjects*, in: Nature Genetics 49, 27–35; Rees, E., Kendall, K., Pardinas, A. F., Legge, S. E., Pocklington, A., Escott-Price, V., MacCabe, J. H., Collier, D. A., Holmans, P., O'Donovan, M. C., Owen, M. J., Walters, J. T. R., Kirov, G. (2016): *Analysis of Intellectual Disability Copy Number Variants for Association With Schizophrenia*, in: JAMA Psychiatry 73, 963–969; Stefansson, H., Meyer-Lindenberg, A., Steinberg, S., Magnusdottir, B., Morgen, K., Arnarsdottir, S., Bjornsdottir, G., Walters, G. B., Jonsdottir, G. A., Doyle, O. M., Tost, H., Grimm, O., Kristjansdottir, S., Snorrason, H., Davidsdottir, S. R., Gudmundsson, L. J., Jonsson, G. F., Stefansdottir, B., Helgadottir, I., Haraldsson, M., Jonsdottir, B., Thygesen, J. H., Schwarz, A. J., Didriksen, M., Stensbol, T. B., Brammer, M., Kapur, S., Halldorsson, J. G., Hreidarsson, S., Saemundsen, E., Sigurdsson, E., Stefansson, K. (2014): *CNVs conferring risk of autism or schizophrenia affect cognition in controls*, in: Nature 505, 361–366.

[6] Dudbridge, F. (2013): *Power and predictive accuracy of polygenic risk scores*, in: PLoS Genetics 9, e1003348.

[7] Schizophrenia Working Group of the Psychiatric Genomics, C. (2014): *Biological insights from 108 schizophrenia-associated genetic loci*, in: Nature 511, 421–427.

ily history, social adjustment, neuropsychological data, and imaging markers, are taken into account.[8]

However, this prediction is probabilistic in nature and can never be specific for a given psychiatric disorder, as defined according to current classification systems (see below: "Shortcomings of Current Diagnoses"). Carriers of the rare schizophrenia-associated CNVs have a much higher risk of developmental delay and/or cognitive deficits than for schizophrenia itself. In addition, increased polygenic risk scores for schizophrenia are not schizophrenia-specific, but are associated with various other conditions and factors, such as other psychiatric disorders[9]; response to medication and disease course[10]; cognitive functioning[11]; social cognition[12]; and brain structure and brain functioning[13].

---

[8] Abi-Dargham, A., Horga, G. (2016): *The search for imaging biomarkers in psychiatric disorders*, in: Nature Medicine 22, 1248–1255.

[9] McGrath, J. J., Mortensen, P. B., Visscher, P. M., Wray, N. R. (2013): *Where GWAS and epidemiology meet: opportunities for the simultaneous study of genetic and environmental risk factors in schizophrenia*, in: Schizophrenia Bulletin 39, 955–959.

[10] Frank, J., Lang, M., Witt, S. H., Strohmaier, J., Rujescu, D., Cichon, S., Degenhardt, F., Nothen, M. M., Collier, D. A., Ripke, S., Naber, D., Rietschel, M. (2015): *Identification of increased genetic risk scores for schizophrenia in treatment-resistant patients*, in: Molecular Psychiatry 20, 150–151.

[11] Benca, C. E., Derringer, J. L., Corley, R. P., Young, S. E., Keller, M. C., Hewitt, J. K., Friedman, N. P. (2017): *Predicting Cognitive Executive Functioning with Polygenic Risk Scores for Psychiatric Disorders*, in: Behavioral Genetics 47, 11–24.

[12] Germine, L., Robinson, E. B., Smoller, J. W., Calkins, M. E., Moore, T. M., Hakonarson, H., Daly, M. J., Lee, P. H., Holmes, A. J., Buckner, R. L., Gur, R. C., Gur, R. E. (2016): *Association between polygenic risk for schizophrenia, neurocognition and social cognition across development*, in: Translational Psychiatry 6, e924.

[13] Erk, S., Mohnke, S., Ripke, S., Lett, T. A., Veer, I. M., Wackerhagen, C., Grimm, O., Romanczuk-Seiferth, N., Degenhardt, F., Tost, H., Mattheisen, M., Muhleisen, T. W., Charlet, K., Skarabis, N., Kiefer, F., Cichon, S., Witt, S. H., Nothen, M. M., Rietschel, M., Heinz, A., Meyer-Lindenberg, A., Walter, H. (2017): *Functional neuroimaging effects of recently discovered genetic risk loci for schizophrenia and polygenic risk profile in five RDoC subdomains*, in: Translational Psychiatry 7, e997; Kauppi, K., Westlye, L. T., Tesli, M., Bettella, F., Brandt, C. L., Mattingsdal, M., Ueland, T., Espeseth, T., Agartz, I., Melle, I., Djurovic, S., Andreassen, O. A. (2015): *Polygenic risk for schizophrenia associated with working memory-related prefrontal brain activation in patients with schizophrenia and healthy controls*, in: Schizophrenia Bulletin 41, 736–743; Ranlund, S., Calafato, S., Thygesen, J. H., Lin, K., Cahn, W., Crespo-Facorro, B., de Zwarte, S. M. C., Diez, A., Di Forti, M., Group, Iyegbe, C., Jablensky, A., Jones, R., Hall, M. H., Kahn, R., Kalaydjieva, L., Kravariti, E., McDonald, C., McIntosh, A. M., McQuillin, A., Peic, Picchioni, M., Prata, D. P., Rujescu, D., Schulze, K., Shaikh, M., Toulopoulou, T., van Haren, N., van Os, J., Vassos, E., Walshe, M., Wtccc, Lewis, C., Murray, R. M., Powell, J., Bramon, E. (2018): *A polygenic risk score analysis of psychosis endophenotypes across brain functional, structural, and cognitive domains*, in: American Journal of Medical Genetics Part B: Neuropsychiatric Genetics 177, 21–34.

Shortcomings of Current Diagnoses

These broad and non-specific association findings are not unexpected. Rather, they are inherent to the shortcomings of classification systems: Between the late nineteenth century and the second half of the 20th century, psychiatrists paid scant attention to diagnosis due to an emphasis on the psychoanalytic approach. Only then did clinicians begin to label psychiatric disorders as particular diagnostic entities, and adopt a medical model of psychiatry.[14] Today, in the absence of any objective biological markers, diagnoses listed in current classification systems are assigned when a defined number of specified symptoms are present for a specified time period. One of the major limitations of current diagnostic systems is that they are simultaneously too broad and too narrow. They are too broad in the sense that patients with the same diagnosis may display differences in terms of symptom constellation and disease-course, and too narrow in the sense that differing psychiatric disorders show symptom overlap. Thus patients with the same clinical diagnosis may have differing aetiologies, while patients with differing diagnoses may have common, or even identical, aetiological factors.

The Need for Large Samples with Refined Characterisation

In consequence, to identify true correlations between clinical and genetic factors, very large datasets and refined characterisation are required. The respective analyses must also take into account findings from neuroimaging and neuropsychological assessments. The establishment of such large samples requires collaboration between many sites. For the phenotype characterization researchers are required to achieve consensus as to which of the many neuropsychological phenotypes represent causal factors, and how these could be assessed in a comparable and standardised manner across study sites. This is a complex undertaking. For example, brain imaging machines and rating instruments must be harmonised, and even an issue as simple as the definition of age-at-onset can prove problematic, since it depends on whether first symptoms, first treatment, or the first episode to fulfill diagnostic criteria is being referred to. Restrictions in budgets, personnel, and of the physical and psychological stamina of study participants impose further limitations on the phenotyping process. The assessment of psychiatric cohorts is thus highly resource and time-intensive, and cannot be carried out within the context of routine clinical practice, rendering well characterised research cohorts a valuable but expensive resource. To justify the intense input required of

---

[14] Aboraya, A., France, C., Young, J., Curci, K., Lepage, J. (2005): *The Validity of Psychiatric Diagnosis Revisited: The Clinician's Guide to Improve the Validity of Psychiatric Diagnosis*, in: Psychiatry (Edgmont) 2, 48–55.

study participants, researchers, and tax payers, these cohorts should be used for as long as they continue to serve the intended research purpose. Such a long-term use is intended for most psychiatric genetic cohorts collected to date. The future use however, depends on the informed consent which has been obtained from the study participant (see below: "Informed Consent").

The IMAGEMEND Project

Since its outset, a major aim of IMAGEMEND has been to establish Europe's largest, integrated imaging, genetic, environmental risk, and clinical database. The overarching aims of the IMAGEMEND project are to: 1) improve both knowledge of the aetiology of mental illness and clinical management through the discovery of neuroimaging-based diagnostic-, trans-diagnostic-, and predictive markers; and 2) facilitate the translation of these markers into clinical diagnostics and therapeutics. To achieve this, the IMAGEMEND consortium is pursuing the following goals:

(a) identification and validation of integrative markers (imaging, genetics, clinical, environmental) for the differential diagnosis of schizophrenia, bipolar disorder, ADHD, and control status;

(b) identification and validation of integrative markers for the prediction of treatment response, relapse, and side effects;

(c) translation of findings to the pre-symptomatic phase in order to identify illness conversion and allow personalised treatment recommendations in patients at risk for major mental disorders, and prediction of persistence of adolescent illness into adulthood.

Ultimately, the results obtained from the IMAGEMEND project will be translated into automated, clinically applicable diagnostic and predictive tests.

The consortium comprises a total of 14 partners from 4 EU and 3 EU-associated countries. The EU partners are based in Germany, Italy, the Netherlands, and the UK. The remaining partners are based in Iceland, Norway, and Switzerland. All IMAGEMEND partner institutions are internationally renowned, and have distinguished track records in psychiatric neuroimaging- and genetic research. The IMAGEMEND project focuses on schizophrenia, bipolar disorder, and ADHD, and has assembled the largest combined neuroimaging, genetic, environmental, cognitive, and clinical dataset in Europe to date. These data have been collected from approximately 13,000 participants. In addition, the IMAGEMEND consortium has access to international replication datasets, which have been collected from more than 30,000 individuals.[15]

---

[15] Imagemend (2018): The IMAGEMENT Study. URL http://www.imagemend.eu/the-imagemend-study-3/the-imagemend-study [15 March 2018].

Ethical Challenges Encountered in the IMAGEMEND Project

Within IMAGEMEND, an ethics workpackage (WP Ethics) has been established in order to address ethical concerns associated with the development and application of novel predictive biomarkers and predictive psychiatric testing for mental illness. The work of WP Ethics involves: a.) scrutiny of all informed consent documentation and procedures; and b.) assessment of the attitudes and ethical viewpoints of patients, relatives, health care professionals, individuals from the general population, and experts from the fields of medical genetics, philosophy, bioethics, theology, and the social sciences with respect to genetic predictive testing, and their precise understanding of the results and the perceived benefit of such risk predictions.

A.) Informed Consent

Informed consent must take into account the autonomy of the individual and the issue of data protection (e.g. the exchange of clinical data and biomaterials with other researchers, or their deposition in public data bases). The informed consent procedure must also address the right of the individual to know, or not to know, about research findings. This issue is of particular importance in the context of Incidental Findings (see below: "incidental findings").[16] From an ethical perspective, these issues are especially complex in the case of individuals who are unable to provide informed consent, e.g. legal minors. Furthermore, among individuals with psychiatric disorders, the likelihood of encountering persons who may be especially vulnerable and/or prone to misunderstanding information is increased. This is compounded by the fact that in some mental disorders, mental states tend to be unstable, and may show rapid and substantial fluctuations over time.

Given that technological progress in the field of genetics is rapid and unforeseeable, broad consent is advisable. This should allow comprehensive and long-term data use, since apart from their scientific quality, the value of the collected data and biomaterials is dependent on how widely they can be applied. Here, the question arises as to whether it is actually possible to provide potential study participants with adequate information concerning future analyses involving as yet unforeseen new technologies. Unexpected results are inherent to research, and given the rapid pace of technological advance in the field of medical (and psychiatric) genetics, researchers must be aware of the fact that they are unlikely to foresee all possible developments. For example, for a long time many researchers

---

[16] Lanzerath, D., Heinrichs, B., Rietschel, M., Schmäl, C. (eds.) (2014): *Incidental Findings: Scientific, Legal and Ethical Issues*, Medizin-Ethik, Bd. 26, Köln.

had not considered that it could become possible to reconstruct individual physiognomy on the basis of genetic data, a development which could jeopardise privacy.[17]

The main challenge therefore is to inform study participants as precisely as possible of: (i) the overall aim of the study; (ii) how – and with what methods – the researchers aim to achieve their goals; (iii) potential risks; and (iv) precautions undertaken to avoid risks, and the potential limitations thereof. A further complication is that an informed consent document which is broad enough to cover all of these uncertainties may not be considered valid. It has been suggested that researchers should re-contact study participants in order to obtain further informed consent when new aspects, not unequivocally covered by the original informed consent, emerge. The concept of a continuous exchange between researchers and study participants is desirable, as it acknowledges the position of the study participant as a partner in the research project, and allows the disclosure of results that may arise at a future time-point during the ongoing analyses if the study participant so wishes.[18] Continuous exchange also provides the researcher with the opportunity to perform long-term follow-up, and to return to study participants who display specific genetic or clinical features for more in depth investigation. For practical reasons, such an approach is often unfeasible in large, long-term multinational studies involving data from many tens of thousands of participants, although this might be resolved if the necessary resources were made available. If re-contact is not an option, researchers could also consider presenting the specific case to the local ethics committee in order to seek their advice as to whether the new aspect/approach is consistent with the original informed consent of the study participant, albeit not explicitly.

To obtain wide-ranging authorisation, WP Ethics suggested that study participants of IMAGEMEND should be informed as follows:

"However, at the present time we are unable to specify the exact research objectives. You should be aware that in consenting to participate in this study, you are granting us very wide-ranging authorisation. Therefore, we request explicit consent to this wide-ranging authorisation, which you can indicate by ticking the respective boxes on the informed consent document."

---

[17] Lippert, C., Sabatini, R., Maher, M. C., Kang, E. Y., Lee, S., Arikan, O., Harley, A., Bernal, A., Garst, P., Lavrenko, V., Yocum, K., Wong, T., Zhu, M., Yang, W. Y., Chang, C., Lu, T., Lee, C. W. H., Hicks, B., Ramakrishnan, S., Tang, H., Xie, C., Piper, J., Brewerton, S., Turpaz, Y., Telenti, A., Roby, R. K., Och, F. J., Venter, J. C. (2017): *Identification of individuals by trait prediction using whole-genome sequencing data*, in: Proceedings of the National Academy of Sciences of the U S A 114, 10166–10171.

[18] Lazaro-Munoz, G., Farrell, M. S., Crowley, J. J., Filmyer, D. M., Shaughnessy, R. A., Josiassen, R. C., Sullivan, P. F. (2018): *Improved ethical guidance for the return of results from psychiatric genomics research*, in: Molecular Psychiatry 23, 15–23.

WP Ethics also advised IMAGEMEND partners concerning the informing of participants about potential risks as e.g. those relating to data protection:

"The collection, storage, and transmission of data obtained from your biomaterials for research projects all carry the risk of a breach of confidentiality (i.e. the possibility exists that you may be identified). This applies in particular to information concerning your genetic material. These risks cannot be completely ruled out, and they increase as possibilities for linking data together increase, e.g. if you yourself publish your genetic data on the Internet (i.e. for genealogical research). [...] Following an appropriate application, the double encrypted biomaterials and medical data can be passed on to other universities, research institutes, or research companies – if necessary abroad – under pre-established criteria for medical research. Under certain circumstances, the data may be linked with medical data sets in other databases, provided that the necessary legal requirements are met. Under certain circumstances, the data may be disclosed to research projects abroad with potentially lower standards of data protection."

To harmonise informed consent across IMAGEMEND sites, WP Ethics formulated a template informed consent document. Project partners were then advised to use this as the basis for drafting their own informed consent documentation, taking into consideration national law and customs, for submission to their local ethics committees. This informed consent template was an adaptation of the *"Template for the donation, storage, and use of biomaterials as well as the collection, processing and use of data in biobanks"*[19] and the *"Template proband information and informed consent documentation for the genetic analysis of samples from adult persons with legal capacity"*[20]. At that time, no English translation was available for use as a 1:1 blueprint for all EU countries, since the formulation is based on German law and the text is written from a German ethics perspective. However, in response to multiple requests, an English translation has meanwhile been made available (performed 20.07.2015).[21] The value of such a blueprint, which facilitates harmonisation and discussion among researchers in Europe, cannot be overestimated, and the credit for this development must be given to the European Network of Research Ethics Committees (EUREC). The blueprint is also of value to clinicians who are attempting to recruit their patients

---

[19] Permanent Working Party of the German Medical Ethics Committees (2013): *Template for the Donation, Storage and Utilization of Biological Materials as well as the Collecting, Processing and Usage of (related) Data in Biobanks*, in: Recommendation approved by General Assembly, 09.11.2013. URL www.ak-med-ethik-komm.de/docs/MustertextBiobanken.docx [24.01.2018].

[20] Permanent Working Party of the German Medical Ethics Committees (2010): *Template for the Patient Information, and Informed Consent for Genetic Analysis of Samples of Adult Persons who are Capable to Consent*, in: Recommendation approved by General Assembly, 27.11.2010. URL https://www.laekh.de/images/Aerzte/Rund_ums_Recht/Ethikkommission/Mustertext_Pat Info_genetisch.pdf [25 January 2018].

[21] The translation can be found at: http://www.ak-med-ethik-komm.de/index.php?option=com_content&view=article&id=145&Itemid=154&lang=de [19 March 2018].

for research projects, since it covers key issues which may be prerequisite in terms of joining international efforts. The blueprint also facilitates discussions with local ethic committees.

Despite the comprehensive coverage of the proposed informed consent documentation, *"the devil is in the detail"*. WP Ethics therefore anticipates challenges during the actual course or the research, such as issues relating to data protection and the disclosure of incidental findings.

Data Protection

As pointed out above, broad use by many researchers will secure the most successful exploitation of the data. To date, adherence to state-of-the-art data protection rules has allowed the relatively uncomplicated exchange of clinical data and biomaterials between European partners.

Exchange of IMAGEMEND data with countries with lower levels of data protection, such as the USA or China, is also possible, provided that study participants have been informed and provide consent. However, a degree of uncertainty has been introduced by the EU General Data Protection Regulation and Directive, which was adopted by the European Parliament in April 2016 and which will come into force on 25 May 2018. Most researchers are uncertain of the implications of this legislation, and whether the informed consent must now be adapted in order to avoid the loss of data for further analyses.

A further point in relation to data protection concerns the transfer of data for extended computational analyses, since new biostatistical methods render the handling of large data sets unpractical/impossible on local computers. Increasingly, use of these methods will require the transfer of data to servers in other countries or continents. For example, the effective imputation, i.e. the statistical inference of genotypes, of large genetic data sets using the most recent reference panels requires the uploading of data to servers in the UK or the USA, as the respective reference panels are not publicly available.[22] Even if the data are deleted immediately after imputation, they are transferred to a non-EU country.

Incidental Findings

Incidental findings have been defined as unexpected observations of potential clinical significance. In psychiatric genetic studies, such findings may arise from several sources, e.g. from the assessment of psychopathology, environmental factors,

---

[22] McCarthy, S., Das, S., Kretzschmar, W., Delaneau, O., Wood, A. R., Teumer, A., Kang, H. M., Fuchsberger, C., Danecek, P., Sharp, K., Luo, Y., Sidore, C., Kwong, A., Timpson, N., Koskinen, S., Vrieze, S., Scott, L. J., Zhang, H., Mahajan, A., Veldink, J., Peters, U., Pato, C., van Duijn,C. M., Gillies, C. E., Gandin, I., Mezzavilla, M., Gilly, A., Cocca, M., Traglia, M.,

neuroimaging data, or genetics. Given that certain events occur at a substantial frequency, the term secondary rather than incidental may be more appropriate. In either case, discussion of the potential for such a finding must be included in the informed consent process. If the frequency of a particular event is known, the chance of detecting the event should be discussed. Given the large number of potential secondary findings, it may also be advisable to determine in advance which type of secondary finding should be disclosed (e.g. only those of clinical relevance, or for which therapeutic or preventive measures can be taken). In all cases, the researcher should explain to the participant that the absence of a finding does not exclude the existence of pathology. Misconceptions concerning further management of any secondary findings should also be identified and clarified in advance. For example, what legitimate expectations can a non-remunerated study participant have of a researcher in this respect? Do these expectations differ if the researcher is also a clinician, who therefore has a professional duty of care? While some degree of consensus has been reached on how to proceed with secondary findings in brain imaging and psychopathology, the situation with respect to genetic testing is a matter of ongoing debate as reviewed by Knoppers and colleagues[23], and Lazaro-Munoz and colleagues.[24]

There is a broad consensus among researchers and clinicians that in order to be disclosed, genetic research results should be both: (i) analytically and clinically valid; and (ii) medically relevant and/or actionable. However, reported opinions range from the disclosure of all genomic information (such as providing test persons with raw data which they may process on their own), to the provision of no individual genetic information at all.

Angius, A., Barrett, J. C., Boomsma, D., Branham, K., Breen, G., Brummett, C. M., Busonero, F., Campbell, H., Chan, A., Chen, S., Chew, E., Collins, F. S., Corbin, L. J., Smith, G. D., Dedoussis, G., Dorr, M., Farmaki, A. E., Ferrucci, L., Forer, L., Fraser, R. M., Gabriel, S., Levy, S., Groop, L., Harrison, T., Hattersley, A., Holmen, O. L., Hveem, K., Kretzler, M., Lee, J. C., McGue, M., Meitinger, T., Melzer, D., Min, J. L., Mohlke, K. L., Vincent, J. B., Nauck, M., Nickerson, D., Palotie, A., Pato, M., Pirastu, N., McInnis, M., Richards, J. B., Sala, C., Salomaa, V., Schlessinger, D., Schoenherr, S., Slagboom, P. E., Small, K., Spector, T., Stambolian, D., Tuke, M., Tuomilehto, J., Van den Berg, L. H., Van Rheenen, W., Volker, U., Wijmenga, C., Toniolo, D., Zeggini, E., Gasparini, P., Sampson, M. G., Wilson, J. F., Frayling, T., de Bakker, P. I., Swertz, M. A., McCarroll, S., Kooperberg, C., Dekker, A., Altshuler, D., Willer, C., Iacono, W., Ripatti, S., Soranzo, N., Walter, K., Swaroop, A., Cucca, F., Anderson, C. A., Myers, R. M., Boehnke, M., McCarthy, M. I., Durbin, R., Haplotype Reference, C. (2016): *A reference panel of 64,976 haplotypes for genotype imputation*, in: Nature Genetics 48, 1279–1283.

[23] Lazaro-Munoz, G., Farrell, M. S., Crowley, J. J., Filmyer, D. M., Shaughnessy, R. A., Josiassen, R. C., Sullivan, P. F. (2018): *Improved ethical guidance for the return of results from psychiatric genomics research*, in: Molecular Psychiatry 23, 15–23.

[24] Knoppers, B. M., Zawati, M. H., Senecal, K. (2015): *Return of genetic testing results in the era of whole-genome sequencing*, in: Nature Reviews Genetics 16, 553–559.

New technologies now allow the detection of pathogenic mutations via rapid genome-wide sequencing. Knowledge of the presence of such a mutation may assist the test person in terms of lifestyle choices or decisions regarding medical screening/care for the test person, and there is ongoing discussion in the medical genetics field as to whether a routine inspection for a list of selected medically actionable genes should be performed during the research process. At the time of writing, this list comprises 59 genes.[25] In this event, the researcher would be required to inform the study participant about this testing, and the many potential test results, during the informed consent process. Furthermore, the consequences would have to be considered if the study participant does not wish to be informed about some (potentially life-threatening) information. In a research setting, this would be a complicated undertaking. In general, the aim of genetic research is to search for hitherto unknown genetic risk factors, rather than to test research participants for known and clinically validated pathogenic mutations.

As the analysis of genome-wide sequencing data is a complicated process, a straightforward interpretation of the impact of a newly identified variant on health is rare. New, potentially pathological, but hitherto unknown genetic variants are by their very nature unlikely to fulfill the standards required for the disclosure of test results.[26]

Furthermore, a principal problem in genetic research is that the disclosure of genetic findings requires specific expertise. Clinical researchers are not necessarily able to interpret incidental findings accurately, and/or provide adequate counselling. Researchers must therefore be able to forward the respective information to clinicians with the requisite training and expertise who know how to interpret validate and communicate potential findings. Although research projects such as IMAGEMEND generally lack resources for interventions of this nature, this requirement can be met adequately when it concerns only single research participants. However, the question of how to proceed in future investigations, when the

---

[25] Kalia, S. S., Adelman, K., Bale, S. J., Chung, W. K., Eng, C., Evans, J. P., Herman, G. E., Hufnagel, S. B., Klein, T. E., Korf, B. R., McKelvey, K. D., Ormond, K. E., Richards, C. S., Vlangos, C. N., Watson, M., Martin, C. L., Miller, D. T. (2017): *Recommendations for reporting of secondary findings in clinical exome and genome sequencing, 2016 update (ACMG SF v2.0): a policy statement of the American College of Medical Genetics and Genomics*, in: Genetics in Medicine 19, 249–255.

[26] Knoppers, B. M., Zawati, M. H., Senecal, K. (2015): *Return of genetic testing results in the era of whole-genome sequencing*, in: Nature Reviews Genetics 16, 553–559; Matthijs, G., Dierking, A., Schmidtke, J. (2016): *New EuroGentest/ESHG guidelines and a new clinical utility gene card format for NGS-based testing*, in: European Journal of Human Genetics 24, 1; Matthijs, G., Souche, E., Alders, M., Corveleyn, A., Eck, S., Feenstra, I., Race, V., Sistermans, E., Sturm, M., Weiss, M., Yntema, H., Bakker, E., Scheffer, H., Bauer, P., EuroGentest, European Society of Human, G. (2016): *Guidelines for diagnostic next-generation sequencing*, in: European Journal of Human Genetics 24, 2–5.

genome of all study participants will be sequenced, has not yet been answered. Further practical issues arise from the long-term use of data. For example, how should researchers proceed when secondary findings only become apparent after an interval of several years? Who will contact the study participant, and by what means?

Anonymisation of the data set has been an option to avoid those problems. However, anonymisation precludes both the gathering of further information with respect to the study aims, and the informing of participants about imminent health risks. In any case, the new EU General Data Protection Regulation does not forsee this possibility anymore.

B.) Attitudes and Ethical Views of Patients, Relatives, Health Care Professionals, and the General Population towards Predictive and Diagnostic Psychiatric Genetic Testing

On the basis of currently available psychiatric genetic data, the International Society of Psychiatric Genetics (ISPG) does not recommend psychiatric diagnostic testing.[27] The ISPG has advised that when psychiatric genetic testing with health implications becomes available, this should be accompanied by expert genetic counselling, as is the case for all genetic testing with health implications. However, given the pace of progress in the field, genetic testing may soon become reality and patients, persons at risk, and individuals from the general population may wish to be informed of their future risk. Psychiatrists and counsellors must therefore be prepared to assist in the interpretation of these results.

An even more challenging issue is one already encountered in research, namely that participants of studies in which genome-wide genetic data are generated may wish to learn about their risk for psychiatric disorders and/or obtain their data sets in order to explore them independently. The calculation of such an increased risk on the basis of genetic data (e.g. high polygenic risk) is in principle already possible, and the availability of ever richer data sets will enable the generation of increasingly precise predictive information. It is unclear whether study participants will be able to handle such information in a way that it does not affect them adversely. Due to the expanding application of genetic approaches in medical research, requests from participants for such data sets, and the associated ethical problems, will only increase over time, and thus researchers must develop appropriate strategies how to deal with such demands.

---

[27] International Society of Psychiatric Genetics (2017): *Genetic Testing Statement*. URL https://ispg.net/genetic-testing-statement/ [15 March 2018].

From their very beginning, the efforts of the present authors to identify the genetic underpinnings of mental illness have been paralleled by research into the associated ethical issues. In 2003, our group conducted a large population-based survey of attitudes towards psychiatric genetic research.[28] The survey involved more than 3077 individuals from the general population, and representatives from several groups of specific interest, e.g. patients, relatives, psychiatrists, psychologists, geneticists, journalists, and pregnant women. In accordance with previous reports,[29] the results revealed high approval towards psychiatric genetic research and clinical testing across all groups.[30] However, the survey also revealed that around third of those in favour of psychiatric genetic research also had ethical concerns. This differentiated view, or outright ambivalence, concerned multiple aspects of the psychiatric genetic research process, as well as the potential consequences and translation into routine clinical management of the research findings. Given the complexity and multifaceted potential consequences of genetic testing, this reserve is understandable. A major issue in genetic testing is the autonomy of the tested person. While the majority of those surveyed were in favour of autonomous decision making, a substantial proportion of respondents were of the opinion that certain individuals (in particular persons with positions of high responsibly, such as pilots) should be obliged to undergo psychiatric genetic testing. For each investigated aspect of psychiatric genetic testing, the highest degree

---

[28] Strohmaier, J., Witt, S., Flatau, L., Lemme, N., Reitt, M., Rujescu, D., Illes, F., Lanzerath, D., Schulze, T. G., Rietschel, M. (2018): *Psychiatric genetic testing: attitudes towards the right to self-determination and development of a checklist for use in future psychiatric genetic counselling*, (in preparation).

[29] Bui, E. T., Anderson, N. K., Kassem, L., McMahon, F. J. (2014): *Do participants in genome sequencing studies of psychiatric disorders wish to be informed of their results? A survey study*, in: PLoS One 9, e101111; Laegsgaard, M. M., Kristensen, A. S., Mors, O. (2009): *Potential consumers' attitudes toward psychiatric genetic research and testing and factors influencing their intentions to test*, in: Genetic Testing and Molecular Biomarkers 13, 57–65; Lawrence, R. E., Appelbaum, P. S. (2011): *Genetic testing in psychiatry: a review of attitudes and beliefs*, in: Psychiatry 74, 315–331; Middleton, A., Morley, K. I., Bragin, E., Firth, H. V., Hurles, M. E., Wright, C. F., Parker, M., study, D. D. D. (2016): *Attitudes of nearly 7000 health professionals, genomic researchers and publics toward the return of incidental results from sequencing research*, in: European Journal of Human Genetics 24, 21–29; Sanderson, S. C., Linderman, M. D., Suckiel, S. A., Diaz, G. A., Zinberg, R. E., Ferryman, K., Wasserstein, M., Kasarskis, A., Schadt, E. E. (2016): *Motivations, concerns and preferences of personal genome sequencing research participants: Baseline findings from the HealthSeq project*, in: European Journal of Human Genetics 24, 14–20; Wilde, A., Meiser, B., Mitchell, P. B., Hadzi-Pavlovic, D., Schofield, P.R. (2011): *Community interest in predictive genetic testing for susceptibility to major depressive disorder in a large national sample*, in: Psychological Medicine 41,1605–1613.

[30] Illes, F. (2008): *Einstellung zu und Risikowahrnehmung bei prädiktiven genetischen Tests bei neuro-psychiatrischen Erkrankungen (Online publizierte Dissertation)*, Rheinische Friedrich-Wilhelms-Universität Bonn. URL hss.ulb.uni-bonn.de/2008/1315/1315.pdf; details in English provided in the supplement [25 January 2018].

of reserve was found among psychiatrists. This suggests that ethical reservations concerning psychiatric genetic testing are dependent upon the degree of expert knowledge or background, and that psychiatrists may foresee problems that are not immediately apparent to other groups. Similarly, patients and relatives may have insights or perspectives that are not evident to psychiatrists. Differing perspectives, backgrounds, or levels of knowledge may thus lead to differing attitudes, and these differences must be taken into account once psychiatric genetic testing in the routine clinical practice setting becomes feasible.

Within the context of IMAGEMEND, the present authors conducted a second survey[31] of attitudes towards psychiatric genetic testing among patients, relatives, and experts. Rather than determining representative numbers, e.g. how many respondents were in favour or against a particular aspect of psychiatric genetic testing, the major aim of the second survey was to explore context-dependent controversies and ambivalence. The results can inform future strategies for the management of study participants who wish to learn more about their research results, and will assist clinicians in the future psychiatric genetic counselling setting by highlighting areas requiring detailed pre- and post-testing discussion.

The second survey focused on controversial topics identified in the 2003 survey, such as the right to self-determination, in order to elucidate whether they were dependent on either the particular context (e.g. preventable and treatable disease), or the specific group in question pilots, children. Case-vignettes were then designed to illustrate the most controversial issues, and these were discussed in a series of Delphi rounds (the Delphi round process is depicted in Figure 1, and an exemplary case-vignette is provided). The findings of the second survey indicate that in psychiatric genetic testing, personal context and values play a role in informed decision-making. Data from the second survey were used to compile a checklist of the most important issues for discussion with an individual who is considering psychiatric genetic testing. This checklist is depicted in Figure 2. The checklist is designed to facilitate informed and autonomous decision-making on the part of the test person. The checklist can be used by researchers when participants wish to discuss their research results, and by clinicians in the future genetic counselling process. If direct-to-consumer psychiatric genetic tests become available, a modified version of the checklist could also be consulted by individuals prior to purchase. In essence, the checklist covers issues that should be considered by anyone who is considering genetic testing. It must be emphasised that the checklist is preliminary, and will require continuous revision as new genetic and functional data and feedback from the future counselling setting become available.

---

[31] Strohmaier, J., Witt, S., Flatau, L., Lemme, N., Reitt, M., Rujescu, D., Illes, F., Lanzerath, D., Schulze, T. G., Rietschel, M. (in preparation).

Conclusion

Psychiatric genetic research promises to elucidate the aetiology of mental disorders, and facilitate the development of future individualised therapies and prevention strategies. Given the complexity of psychiatric genetic data, all individuals who participate in genetic testing in either the research or clinical setting should receive adequate information concerning the possible implications of the generated data. Ideally, testing should be performed in the context of a pre- and post-test genetic counselling process.[32] In this counselling process, the reasons for undergoing genetic testing, the potential for incidental and secondary findings and for data of unknown significance, and the associated potential for anxiety and uncertainty, should be discussed with the test person – as well as with all potentially at-risk relatives – both *before and after* the testing procedure. At first glance, an intensive genetic counselling process of this nature may seem too resource intensive for application in routine clinical practice. Alternatively, the handling of psychiatric genetic findings could prove to be as straightforward as the handling of any other routine clinical finding. Biologically valid diagnoses, well replicated genetic association findings, and the establishment of evaluation algorithms may render the interpretation of genetic findings and their integration into clinical routine diagnostics a simpler matter than currently anticipated.

---

[32] International Society of Psychiatric Genetics (2017): *Genetic Testing Statement*. URL https://ispg.net/genetic-testing-statement/ [15 March 2018].

Delphi Process

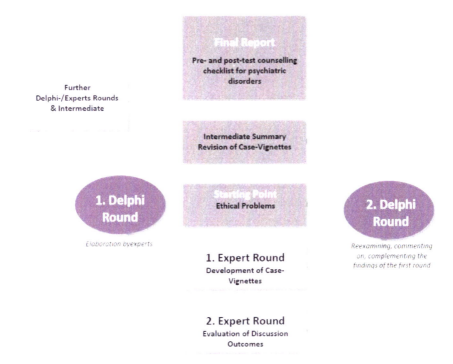

Figure 1: Delphi Process Schematic

Case Vignettes

WP Ethics has now discussed a total of 7 case vignettes in several Delphi rounds. The example pertaining specifically to research in minors is presented below.

Case Vignette #1: Genetic testing in children

Schizophrenia is a severe mental illness characterised by profound disturbances of thought, perception, and emotion. Frequent symptoms are delusions and hallucinations, as well as a flattening of emotion and a lack of drive. To assign a diagnosis of schizophrenia, the symptoms must have been present for at least six months.

Psychiatric genetic research has identified a number of copy-number variations (CNVs). To varying degrees, these CNVs increase the risk for developing schizophrenia. CNVs are a form of structural variation of the DNA of a genome, which results in a variation in the number of copies of one or more sections of the cellular DNA. For certain genes, these changes are non-pathological. CNVs correspond to relatively large regions of the genome that have been either deleted (fewer than the normal number of copies) or duplicated (more than the normal number of copies) on certain chromosomes.

An individual who carries a CNV is at increased risk for schizophrenia. However, as the increase in risk is also dependent on other factors, this individual may remain completely healthy or develop other non-specific psychiatric symptoms or disorders, e.g. depression.

A 49-year old father consulted his family doctor because over the past year, the academic performance of his 12-year old son had steadily declined. His son had performed well in elementary school, and had experienced no problems with the transition to secondary school. Up until the previous year, he had been well integrated, had had many friends, and had had no problems with his teachers. However, within the preceding 12 months, he had become increasingly isolated, and now preferred to play alone at home rather than meeting with friends. The father reported that his son often just sat around staring into space. His academic performance had shown a dramatic decline, with a one point drop in his grades.

The father was aware that he is himself was carrier of a rare CNV that has been reported to increase the risk for schizophrenia. He suffered occasional non-specific depressive symptoms, but was otherwise healthy. However, his sister, who carried the same CNV, had been diagnosed with schizophrenia at the age of 32.

The father explained that he would like his son to undergo testing for the rare CNV. He wished to know whether his son was a carrier in order to guide his approach to his son's difficulties. He stated that if his son proved to have the rare CNV, he would shield him from stress; whereas if he was not a carrier, he would have to search for other reasons for his son's behaviour or insist upon an improvement in his academic and social performance.

The son refused to undergo testing. He stated that his parents annoyed him, and that he did not want to be stigmatised.

Questions

– Should the father be legally entitled to have his son tested?
– Should the father be allowed to have his son tested without his son's knowledge?
– What if the son were 9 years old?
– Would testing be acceptable if the son was in agreement?

Discussion of Case Vignette #1: Genetic Testing in Children

Dr. Kevin McGhee (Acting Deputy Dean Education & Professional Practice, Associate Professor in Health sciences – Faculty of Science & Technology, Bournemouth University, Dorset, UK) pointed out that in this case, the genetic test is not required to indicate that the child is at risk, since there is a known family history. The decision as to whether or not to protect the child from stress may thus be made without genetic testing. Professor Ole Mors (Department of Clinical Medicine, Aarhus University, Aarhus, Denmark) cautioned that the father is jumping too quickly to the assumption that his son may have schizophrenia. Ole Mors said that in the first instance, the child requires assessment by a child psychiatrist, as he may be suffering from another form of psychiatric disturbance, e.g. depression. He emphasised that standard clinical assessment and management must not be bypassed just because a genetic test is available. The child's problems should be defined, and the child should receive help regardless of the potential presence of a copy number variant (CNV). Ole Mors said that in the case of a false positive finding, the identification through genetic testing of a CNV may result in stigmatisation and unnecessary treatment in a child who would never have developed schizophrenia. Professor Dan Rujescu (MD, Director – Department of Psychiatry, Psychotherapy, and Psychosomatics, Martin-Luther-University, Halle, Germany) pointed out that the assumption of 100% penetrance is incorrect. Professor Nick Martin (Queensland Institute of Medical Research Berghofer Medical Research Institute, Brisbane, Australia) added that we not know whether the CNV is causal, especially since the father carries the CNV but does not have the disease. Professor Thomas Schulze (MD, Director- Institute of Psychiatric Phenomics and Genomics, Ludwig-Maximilans-University, Munich, Germany) commented that this vignette provides little detailed information about the family history, and that he would like to have information on the extended pedigree in order to improve his understanding of the perspective of the father and his reasons for wanting the test performed. However, he and Professor Francis McMahon (MD, Principal Investigator – Human Genetics Branch, National Institute of Mental Health, National Institutes of Health, Bethesda, USA) both agreed that this information, e.g. the finding that there was a strong family history of schizophrenia, would not actually influence the decision as to whether the test was indicated in this particular case. Nick Martin pointed out that the son does not want the test, and that enforcing it might therefore damage the father-son relationship. Francis McMahon agreed that in insisting on the performance of the test, the father could be risking more than would be gained through obtaining the test result, and that the son could be left in a situation where he would have to deal, for the rest of his life, with the knowledge of genetic information he had not wanted to receive in the first place. Francis McMahon pointed out that the genetic test may also give rise to other problems, e.g. a secondary finding. Professor Markus Nöthen (MD, Director – Institute of Human Genetics; Department of Genomics, Life & Brain Center, University of Bonn, Bonn, Germany) said that a distinction must be made between diagnostic and predictive testing, and that in view of the child's clinical presentation in this vignette, the issue here relates to diagnostic rather than predictive testing. Markus Nöthen said that in Germany, the criteria for diagnostic testing are relaxed compared to those for predictive testing. However, even for diagnostic testing, the availability of evidence based data is an important prerequisite for performing the genetic test, and that genetic testing is only useful if it will influence the clinical management of the patient. Markus Nöthen said that as he understood it, the clinical management in this case would be entirely dependent upon the phenotype, and that genetic data would not influence management. As a result, in his opinion there is no justification for performing the test.

Professor Christina M. Hultman (Department of Medical Epidemiology and Biostatistics, Karolinska Institute, Stockholm, Sweden) added that at present, no adequate genetic prediction for schizophrenia is available, and that we do not know how environmental and genetic risks add up. She also pointed out that the risk in the child remains low and emphasised the risk of stigmatisation through genetic testing.

Professor Marcella Rietschel (MD, Head of Department – Department of Genetic Epidemiology in Psychiatry, Central Institute of Mental Health, Medical Faculty Mannheim, University of Heidelberg, Mannheim, Germany) pointed out that these vignettes will be shown to other target groups, and that previous research has shown that parents do want to know, and that from her clinical experience she assumes that a lot of parents would wish to know the genetic risk in their child. The panel then discussed how they would view the request for testing if the child was in agreement with it. Francis McMahon said that the agreement of the child would have little impact on the decision in this particular case, as it would not change the main reasons against testing. He also said that it would be important to examine the child's capacity to understand the implications of what he is consenting to.

Key Issues Raised by This Vignette

1. Are the assumptions being made by the person who is requesting the test correct?
2. Will the result of the genetic test influence management? Is genetic testing the correct first step?
3. Could the genetic test have potential harmful effects?
4. Will legislation need to change in order to keep pace with advances in predictive/ diagnostic genetic testing?

The consensus of the panel was that in this particular case, no genetic testing should be performed, even if the son was in agreement, since knowledge of his own genetic make-up would deprive him of his future adult right not to know.

Checklist for Psychiatric Genetic Testing

Figure 2: Checklist for psychiatric genetic testing

Checklist

Note: genetic testing must be carried out within the framework of national laws, regulations, and the recommendations of relevant scientific societies. Furthermore, any genetic testing with health implications should be accompanied by expert genetic counselling. This checklist is intended to offer complementary guidance, by listing those issues which medical specialists, patients, and family members have identified as the most important issues to be considered during future psychiatric genetic counselling:

– Purpose of testing
  – Expectations of clinician and test person
– Information about the disorder
  – Nature of the disorder that will be tested for
  – Test person's concept of disease
– Information about the genetic test
  – Nature of the genetic test (analytic and clinical validity)
  – Potential genetic test results
– Topics to consider
  – Confidentiality and data protection
  – Test person lacks legal capacity for informed consent
  – Subjective perception of risk
  – Capacity to understand risk estimates
  – Planning of further procedures
– Potential benefits and risks

For each checklist item, exemplary issues are presented:

Checklist Topic	Exemplary Issues
Purpose of Testing	
Expectations	Although the clinician who proposes genetic testing in the research or clinical context has a clear aim, the expectation of the tested individual may differ. Furthermore, diverse expectations may be encountered among persons considering genetic testing. Healthy individuals may wish to estimate their own risk for a disease, be informed about prevention, or obtain knowledge of relevance to family- and life-planning.

	Persons at increased risk or with unclear symptoms may hope that testing will inform them about their disease risk, or facilitate the assignment of a definite diagnosis. Diseased individuals may wish to be informed about treatment, medication response, side-effects, or disease course. Some individuals may expect to obtain certainty about their risk status and thus psychological relief. Research subjects may wish to receive feedback on their study results in order to learn about their genetic-make up and potential risk status. The clinician must judge whether, and to what extent, the test and the anticipated consequences will meet these expectations. In the counselling process, this must be communicated in an adequate and understandable manner, which balances the complex and potentially conflicting factors of autonomy, beneficence, and nonmaleficence. If genetic testing is required, or research test results are to be disclosed, pre-test and post-test counselling is required. In addition, easily comprehensible summaries of the results must be made available to the test persons.
Information about the Disorder	
Nature of the disorder that will be tested for	Explain the prevalence, and the complexity of the causes and clinical presentation, of the disorder to the test-person. Explain the concept of a complex genetic disorder; recurrence risk; mode of inheritance; and the current level of knowledge with respect to genetic markers (common, rare, de novo markers), and how they may impact the informational value of the test. Inform the test-person that individuals with the same genetic make-up may differ in terms of aetiology, age at onset, disease symptoms, disease severity, and disease course, and – if relevant – that the clinical presentation of a disease can differ widely from that of an affected family member. Discuss whether – and if so which – prevention/treatment measures are available.
Disease concept	Discuss the test-person's understanding of the disease and its causes. For example, the test person may believe that the disease is inherited, caused by a viral infection, attributable to an unhealthy lifestyle, or has been inflicted as a "punishment". Assumptions about the cause of a disease influence how the individual copes with the disease symptoms. Be aware of potential religious and cultural differences in terms of disease concepts and assumed causes.

Information about the Test and Potential Results	
Nature of genetic test	Explain the analytic validity of the test (accuracy, reliability, sensitivity, and specificity), i.e. whether the test accurately and reliably measures what it should measure. Explain the clinical validity of the test (diagnostic specificity and sensitivity, positive and negative predictive values), i.e. how well the test predicts the clinical condition it is intended to measure. Explain that the reported risk conferred by a specific genetic variant is dependent on the population in which it was tested." Discuss how much the test costs, and who will have to pay for it.
Potential genetic test results	To facilitate an informed decision on the part of the test person concerning the disclosure of test results, explain the meaning of: (i) "increased risk', i. e. the impact of the test's prediction certainty; (ii) confidence intervals; (iii) differences in risk estimates depending on the investigated genetic variant; (iv) the potential for secondary findings, depending on the particular genetic test performed (targeted or genome-wide scan); (v) the relevance of secondary findings in terms of prevention or treatment. Explain whether the test investigates common genetic variants with small effects that are combined into a polygenic risk score, or rare genetic variants with stronger effects such as copy-number-variants (CNVs).
	Explain how genetic test information adds to other available information… Explain that the familial constellation, e.g. "several affected family members carry the same rare variant," is relevant in terms of the interpretation of the test results, and enquire whether the same genetic variant has already been investigated in other affected family members. Explain the meaning of "pleiotropic effects" and "reduced penetrance". Consider whether test results may affect further (as yet untested) family members, and discuss the potential implications of the test result for these persons.

Topics to Consider	
Confidentiality and data protection	Enquire who should be informed about any medically relevant findings and discuss the potential consequences of this information, e.g. in terms of life-insurance, stigma. Discuss the potential consequences for further family members.
Persons unable to consent (e.g. minors and acutely ill patients)	If the test-person lacks legal capacity to provide informed consent (e.g. minors) or has an impaired decision making capacity (e.g. is experiencing the acute phase of a psychiatric disorder), a legal representative and the clinician must reach a joint decision as to whether the beneficence of the test outweighs the violation of autonomy. The option of postponing the test until the test-person is able to consent (e.g. a minor becoming legally able to consent or a patient recovering from an acute episode) must also be taken into consideration.
Subjective perception of risk	Keep in mind that subjective risk estimation is a function of mathematical risk and subjective values. Subjective values can be influenced by factors such as personality (e.g. high vs. low monitoring of risk) and disease state.
Capacity to understand risk estimates	Keep in mind that risk estimates are difficult to understand, and that the test person, in particular a patient with a psychiatric disorder, may have cognitive impairments, emotional problems, and disease symptoms which impact their capacity to understand them. Cognitive impairments and emotional problems may also be present in healthy relatives.
Planning of future procedures	Discuss how test results can be used in prevention or treatment Discuss whether additional testing or a further diagnostic procedure is advisable. Depending on the impact of the test results on the test-person's mental state, a follow up counselling session may be necessary.

Potential Benefits and Risks		
Consequences	Discuss	
	Potential Benefits	Potential Risks
	– More precise estimates of disease risk – Knowledge to facilitate life-planning – Psychological relief – Information concerning treatment or prevention	– Despite increased risk, no prevention available – Psychological stress due to increased risk/or misunderstanding of test results – Behavioural changes (e. g. excessive use of health care services, secrecy in the family) – Stigmatisation and discrimination – Implications for insurance policies – Harm in terms of the right of family members not to know (especially minors)

Although psychiatric genetic testing is in its infancy, researchers and clinicians must be prepared for the ethical implications of the advent of predictive and diagnostic psychiatric genetic tests. This checklist provides the clinician with a guideline for the counselling process in order to facilitate comprehensive coverage of the most relevant issues and thus an informed and autonomous decision on the part of the test person.

Use of Population-based Samples in Psychiatric Genetics: Ethical Considerations

Christina M. Hultman, Viktoria Johansson

General Outline

Genetic testing in psychiatry is sensitive and less accepted than in many physical disorders. From the patient's perspective it might be stigmatizing. From the clinician's perspective it might be difficult with diagnostic specificity as there are less clear biological markers related to psychiatric disorders. From the researcher's perspective the knowledge of solid genetic risk factors still is in its infancy. Our research group have over ten years of experience from psychiatric genetic studies in schizophrenia, bipolar disorder, autism and obsessive-compulsive disorder, collecting blood samples from over 15,000 individuals. In the following chapter, we will give some ethical aspects of studies based on national health registers in Sweden.

Swedish Registers that Make Large Population-based Genetic Studies Possible

The Swedish health register's main goal is to capture health statistics for planning and evaluation, but it is also after strict ethical control an important source for researchers who can apply for data. The Swedish Patient register was established in 1973. All hospitals are required to report the final diagnostic ICD code and treatment period to the Swedish National Board of Health and Welfare. Successively since 2005 also outpatient specialist care has been included. This opens up for the possibility to identify all patients treated with a specific psychiatric diagnosis in Sweden through the register. For schizophrenia, we selected those who had been treated as inpatients at least twice to get a better diagnostic validity. About 30% had only one inpatient stay and were excluded. A linkage with the Death Register gave us further information on who was possible to contact.

Register Recruitment Research

To recruit patients from a national register is different from clinical recruitment in many practical and psychological aspects.[1]

To donate blood in a clinical setting is often within a safe doctor-patient relationship. The question to participate in a genetic study does usually not come as surprise for the patient, as the patient often get questions regarding family history in the anamnestic clinical assessments. The patients can ask questions immediately about details and possible outcomes. Usually treatment aspects are connected to the situation. Perception of genetic risks could be discussed within a frame of help-seeking. Further, the patients take for granted that the information will stay in the room or be protected within hospital and study documents.

For register recruitment research, the individual person is entering as a study participant not as a patient. Before contacting the person via participation inquiry letter, we have sought approval from Psychiatric Executive Groups in all Swedish Councils with local information and a study protocol, but the study is not dependent on individual approval from the study person's doctor. We inform them, from where we got their name and about the possibility to make studies after careful ethical approval in national registers. Some participants might not be aware of those registers and it is a frequent question to the nurses who call for follow-up. The diagnosis could be distant in time and the person might be symptom-free with no clinical contact or current treatment. As an individual with a good prognosis also is interesting as a study participant in our genetic studies, we describe in the study information that their participation is welcomed. Sometimes the individuals do not acknowledge they have got for instance a diagnosis of schizophrenia – the doctor's information might not have been clear or the individual lack in insight. This is more difficult to handle. The contacting nurse usually tells the person that they have the right to get information on from where and when they got the diagnosis and that it is of course voluntary to participate.

Table 1:

CLINICAL RESEARCH

- Doctor – Patient relationship
- Proxy in time
- Relevant for treatment
- Risk communication within a frame of help-seeking
- Secrecy easier to understand

---

[1] See Table 1.

Register recruitment research

- Status as a study participant not patient
- Study participant might not be aware of central registers
- The first reaction if contacted often is: Why me? By chance? Or for a particular diagnosis?
- Diagnosis could be a long time ago
- The study participant might not want to acknowledge the diagnosis
- Not always fully informed of diagnosis by the doctor
- Decision to participate independent of care

Current Population-based Genetic Cohorts

We started with a pilot study on cases with schizophrenia in 2005. Between the years 1973 and 2001, the Swedish Patient Registry had over 325,000 hospital admissions registered for 57,000 individuals. 40,000 fulfilled the criteria of two admissions for schizophrenia, 22,000 were alive and about 35% agreed to donate blood. To ascertain controls we approached a random sample from the general population matched on county, age and sex. Interestingly, the willingness to participate in the study was similar among cases and controls. In the table below, we show our latest cohorts. The diagnostic ascertainment may differ between the cohorts, but the ethical aspects and the feedback we have got from study participants are similar.

Table 2:

Our genetic cohorts with national sampling frame:

SCHIZOPHRENIA	2006-2010	5,851 cases
BIPOLAR DISORDER	2009-2012	5,000 cases
INFANTILE AUTISM	2011-	1,100 cases
		250 parents and child ('trios')
		50 grandparents and grandchildren
OCD	2014-	1,100 cases
TWINS WITH SCHIZOPHRENIA		
BIPOLAR DISORDER	2006-2011	380 twins
CONTROLS	2006-2010	7,145 controls

Interview Study of Reasons to Participate in Genetic Testing

Our first 1,000 study participants with a diagnosis of schizophrenia were asked by the contacting research nurse why they choose to donate blood in a genetic study. The answers were very consistent that they wanted to contribute to science and a good sake, help individuals with severe psychiatric diagnoses, contribute to the goal that other persons would not suffer as much as they had and help their children to a better treatment and care. Many participants said they realize that it might not help them personally as science is a long-term process. A few asked the question of getting detailed feedback on their own genetic make-up. In line with our qualitative study on informed consent preferences among individuals at possible risk for cancer, psychiatric study subjects share a concern for low participation rate and low interest in important research questions with the investigator.[2]

Ethical Issues in Collecting and Use of Data

Empirical studies on ethical issues in schizophrenia research consistently show that to help others and help research are the most important reasons to participate, which we could confirm in our questionnaire mentioned above.[3] Patients strongly support schizophrenia research and associate research with a feeling of hope – a perspective that is strongly underestimated by psychiatrists. It has also been shown that psychiatrists underestimate the patient's trust in researchers. An important finding is that patients want to form their own judgement of the protocol and to decide if they want to participate. Thus, the opinion of a treating doctor, of a relative, another care person, or societal representative needs to be balanced against the individual patient's decision to participate in a study. It was explicitly mentioned in the information letter that the study proposal should be sent directly to the individual patient to avoid paternalism. We chose to have a close contact with patient organizations and parents of patients with schizophrenia in our steering groups to assure an open communication.

Current use of data and future use need to be clearly specified in the informed consent letter. Collaboration sites within and outside the EU need to be specified as well as anonymous data repository if used. The issue of specific or broad use by other researchers could be optional with a question in the informed consent '*I*

---

[2] Hultman, C. M., Lindgren, A. C., Hansson, M. G., Carlstedt-Duke, J., Ritzén, M., Persson, I., Kieler, H. (2009): *Ethical issues in cancer register follow-up of hormone treatment in adolescence*, in: Public Health Ethics 2 (1), 30–36.

[3] Roberts, L. W., Warner, T. D., Brody, J. L., Roberts, B., Lauriello, J., Lyketsos C. (2002): *Patient and psychiatrist ratings of hypothetical schizophrenia research protocols: assessment of harm potential and factors influencing participation decisions*, in: The American Journal of Psychiatry 159 (4), 573–584.

accept that my data is used in other studies that are ethically approved'. It is our experience that about 90% of the study participants allow a broader use outside psychiatry. It seems as if when they have come to the conclusion to participate, they are generous towards other scientific use. The ethical committee demands thorough information about the source of psychiatric diagnoses, clear information about variables taken from registries, validated diagnostic information and protection of sensitive information in all stages. Biobank data are strictly regulated with Material Transfer Agreement between institutions and approved ethical consent.

What is Special about Twin Research?

One of our cohorts consists of twins identified via the Swedish Twin Registry linked to the Patient registry. As participation of twin pairs, in which one or both twins have the disease of interest, is essential for a twin study design, the recruitment in pairs is desirable. It was not a condition though and the twins were recruited independently and not conditioned on the other twin's participation. The ethical issues involved contacting the non-affected sibling, who might not be aware of the affected twin's diagnosis. In a qualitative study of non-affected siblings to patients with schizophrenia, we have shown that an important issue in the relationship between siblings is closeness and caring, but also distancing, fear of heredity that contributes to their own psychiatric symptoms and concerns that their children will be affected.[4] We experienced a strong motivation to participate, an altruistic attitude and curiosity from the non-affected twin. We have also experienced a fear of disclosure of similar traits and distancing. Some twin reported that they do not want personal contact with the affected twin, but took part in the study to contribute with something good for the sibling. As we approached adult twins, many had lived geographically and psychologically very far from each other and there were in many cases moving reconnections.

ETHICAL ASPECTS OF TWIN RECRUITING

– Involvement of non-affected twin
– Balance the right to participate and fear of disclosure
– Monozygotic non-affected twin often curious or distanced
– Altruistic motives
– We have seen many moving reunions

---

[4] Stålberg, G., Ekerwald, H., Hultman, C. M. (2004):*At issue: siblings of patients with schizophrenia: sibling bond, coping patterns, and fear of possible schizophrenia heredity*, in: Schizophrenia Bulletin 30 (2), 445–458.

Feedback of Results and Report of Genetic Deviations

The right to know results from genetic testing in research is frequently being discussed. A debated question is if incidental and secondary findings should be communicated to study participants. The ethical frame differs in different countries and Germany for example has stricter rules than Scandinavia. Most common in psychiatric genetic studies in Sweden is that we state from the beginning that they will not get feedback from the genetic analyses. The aim of the studies and the ethical permission do not include focus on incidental findings of for instance dementia or cancer. In the future, however, when we know more about genetic prediction all over the field it is reasonable to communicate back incidental and secondary findings. In our new schizophrenia collection, we have added a sentence in the informed consent *'If the researchers identify a genetic aberration in my data that gives a major risk increase for a serious modifiable genetic disorder, I want to get information about the results'*. With this question, the right not to know is also met.

What Makes Genetic Testing in Psychiatry so Challenging?

In summary, genetic testing in psychiatry is more challenging in comparison with physical diseases. It is less accepted, more complex, more diverse and more stigmatizing. There are less clear biological markers and the knowledge of genetic risk factors is still in its infancy. In psychiatry there is a high co-morbidity among different diagnoses. Thus, the genetic risk might not be specific to a narrow diagnosis. Recruitment via national registers may differ from clinical recruitment in many practical and ethical details, but the basic needs of an individual to be taken seriously and to be given advice and information at today's level of genetic knowledge, are universal.

Ethics and the Research with Minors – A European Perspective: Challenges of Pediatric Clinical Research

Pirkko LEPOLA

Introduction

The practical challenges of pediatric clinical research can be divided roughly into the two main categories of common life: legal and social. Both of these categories cover the wide spectrum of ethical issues due to the legal, social and developmental status of the minors; vulnerable population with limitations to understand.

The European Union (EU) pediatric population (approx. 100 million children aged 0 to 17 years) is primarily healthy. Therefore, the number of children having certain medical condition is quite limited for each clinical research project, especially for the clinical trials (CT) for new medicinal products. Moreover, children have different forms of diseases than adults, such as very rare diseases or diseases existing only in the childhood.

Despite a rather long history of drug development, there are still not enough studied and safe medicines for children. For that reason, pediatric pharmacotherapy has relied largely on medicines intended for adult use without research data on safety or efficacy, or long-term effects in children.[1] Therefore, international research is necessary to expedite the study of treatments and to bring new beneficial medication to the market for children. This is a general method for safeguarding public health. In 2007, the European Paediatric Regulation (EU 1901/2006) came into force in Europe to support this development.[2] This regulation includes a requirement that the pharmaceutical industry has to conduct CTs with new medicines also on children, if the European Medicines Agency (EMA) and it's Pediatric Committee (PDCO) judges that the medicine is essential and needed in

---

[1] Conroy, S., Choonara, I., Impicciatore, P., Mohn, A., Arnell, H., Rane, A., Knoeppel, C., Seyberth, H., Pandolfini, C., Raffaelli, M. P., Rocchi, F., Bonati, M., Jong, G., de Hoog, M., van den Anker, J. (2000): *Survey of unlicensed and off label drug use in paediatric wards in European countries*, in: BMJ: British Medical Journal 320 (7227), 79–82. URL http://www.ncbi.nlm.nih.gov/pmc/articles/PMC27251/ [31 August 2017].

[2] European Commission (2006): *Regulation (EC) No 1901/2006 of the European Parliament and of the Council of 12 December 2006 on medicinal products for paediatric use and amending Regulation (EEC) No 1768/92, Directive 2001/20/EC, Directive 2001/83/EC and Regulation (EC) No 726/2004*, in: Official Journal of the European Union, 26 January 2007, L 378/1–19. URL http://ec.europa.eu/health/files/eudralex/vol-1/reg_2006_1901/reg_2006_1901_en.pdf [31 August 2017].

that population.[3] This regulation tends to avoid any unnecessary trials in children, but in the near future the number of the needed pediatric CTs eventually increases and complexity emerges, as these are mainly conducted as multinational, multicentre trials due to small patient populations.[4]

Every CT needs a separate Competent Authority (CA) and Ethics Committee (EC) approval in each participating country. The documentation about the research protocol, facilities, research personnel, and general ethical assessment, are part of the submission packages. Pediatric CTs are rather new in the history of clinical research. The unique feature of pediatric clinical research consists of the broad age distribution of the population: from birth to near adulthood, across all therapeutic areas, together with privacy requirements and possible risks, discomfort and expected benefits. This creates demanding research environment for trial design, subject recruitment and trial conduction. The pharmaceutical industry and investigators spend much time and resources preparing the documentation for CA and EC submissions. In Europe, these submissions vary between countries, due to non-harmonized legislation and guidance.

Legal Variations

National Autonomy Leads to Wide Variation in Practice in Europe

As well as European – and international – legislation recognize the age limits for the legal adulthood with the responsibilities and individual authority for the different type of decisions for all spectrum of life, it has created other age-limits below this legal age. The United Nations Convention on the Rights of the Child defines a child as everyone under 18 years unless, *"under the law applicable to the child, majority is attained earlier"*[5]. The national legislation of EU Member States (and non-member states) covers various different age-limits in many sectors, such as

---

[3] European Medicines Agency (2017): *Paediatric Committee (PDCO)*. URL http://www.ema.europa.eu/ema/index.jsp?curl=pages/about_us/general/general_content_000265.jsp&mid=WC0b01ac0580028e9d [31 August 2017].

[4] European Medicines Agency (2012): *5-year Report to the European Commission. General report on the experience acquired as a result of the application of the Paediatric Regulation*. URL http://ec.europa.eu/health/files/paediatrics/2012-09_pediatric_report-annex1-2_en.pdf [31 August 2017]; European Medicines Agency (2016): *10-year Report to the European Commission. General report on the experience acquired as a result of the application of the Paediatric Regulation*. URL https://ec.europa.eu/health/sites/health/files/files/paediatrics/2016_pc_report_2017/ema_10_year_report_for_consultation.pdf[31 August 2017].

[5] United Nations (1990): *Convention on the Rights of the Child. Adopted and opened for signature, ratification and accession by General Assembly resolution 44/25 of 20 November 1989, entry into force 2 September 1990, in accordance with article 49. 1990*. URL http://www.ohchr.org/en/professionalinterest/pages/crc.aspx [31 August 2017].

for driving licenses, independent decisions for medical care, and criminal responsibility. Ever since modern ethical guidelines for medical research in humans[6], it has been a tradition to use protective age limits for children below the legal adulthood, generally 18-years in Europe.

Legal Instruments around Pediatric CTs

The EU regulatory framework for CTs in pediatric population is covered by three legal instruments; the Convention on Human Rights and Biomedicine (the Oviedo Convention)[7], the Paediatric Regulation[8] and the Directive 2001/20/EC (CT Directive)[9]. Of these, the CT Directive has been replaced by the new EU Clinical Trial Regulation [EU No 536/2014] (CTR)[10] in 2014, but it is not yet fully implemented due to the new electronic portal which is still under construction. When fully implemented and used in practice (late 2019), the CTR replaces the CT Directive. The CTR enhances not only the new Clinical Trial Application (CTA) processes by requiring new harmonized procedures regarding to shorter and stricter timelines and reporting, but will also lead to major changes for the EC processes. However, the CTR includes one problem; the overall ethical acceptance will remain with each EU Member State, and cannot be harmonized by the CTR.

Due to national autonomy and national legislation, every European country has created more specific and detailed age limits for children taking part in clinical research and CTs.[11] Furthermore, the details of the national legislation, nor the

---

[6] See Table 1.
[7] Council of Europe (1999): *Convention for the Protection of Human Rights and Dignity of the Human Being with regard to the Application of Biology and Medicine: Convention on Human Rights and Biomedicine*. URL http://conventions.coe.int/Treaty/en/Treaties/Html/164.htm [31 August 2017].
[8] European Commission 2006.
[9] European Commission (2011): *Directive 2001/20/EC of the European Parliament and of the Council of 4 April 2001 on the approximation of the laws, regulations and administrative provisions of the Member Status relating to the implementation of good clinical practice in the conduct of clinical trials on medicinal products for human use*. in: Official Journal of the European Union, 1 May 2001, L 121/34–44. URL https://ec.europa.eu/health/sites/health/files/files/eudralex/vol-1/dir_2001_20/dir_2001_20_en.pdf [31 August 2017].
[10] European Commission (2014): *Regulation (EU) No 536/2014 of the European Parliament and of the Council of 16 April 2014 on clinical trials on medicinal products for human use, and repealing Directive 2001/20/EC*. Official Journal of the European Union, 16 June 2014. URL https://ec.europa.eu/health/sites/health/files/files/eudralex/vol-1/reg_2014_536/reg_2014_536_en.pdf [31 August 2017].
[11] European Network of Paediatric Research at the European Medicines Agency (2017): *Informed Consent and Assent for Paediatric Clinical Trials in Europe 2015*. URL http://tinyurl.com/h2xrlvr [15 January 2018]; Lepola, P., Needham, A., Mendum, J., Sallabank, P., Neubauer, D., de Wildt, S (2016): *Informed Consent for Paediatric Clinical Trials in Europe*, in: Archives of

scientific grounds for these details, have never been discussed properly in Europe across the learned societies, scientific associations, regulators and medical community, in order to reach the harmonized solution. As a result, this has led to great variations between the countries.

Missing Detailed Uniform Guidelines

Pediatric CTs need also very specific design and expertise, suitable facilities and experienced, qualified and trained research personnel. Equally important is the experience of the people designing pediatric research protocols and those reviewing and assessing the protocols; these have to be done according to the high ethical standards and must be scientifically justified.[12]

The international and the ethics societies' guidelines, recommendations and legal texts rarely detail CT related procedures for children, but include often very generic instructions without specific definitions. For the greater part, these criteria do not seem to be based on the developmental stage of the child and his/her competency level. Many of these CT activities are covered by several ethical guidelines, but most of all, by different recommendations. These recommendations are not mandatory requirements allowing different interpretation and implementation in accordance with national legislation. Moreover, it appears that these criteria, for unknown reasons, are not uniformly defined.[13] The latest internationally developed guideline for pediatric medicines is trying to target several of these commonly acknowledged problematic issues seeking to reflect the latest scientific and technical knowledge and provide harmonized updated guidance for pediatric drug development and CTs. This ICH E11(R1) Addendum was under revision and it was finalized in April 2018.[14]

Disease in Childhood 101 (11), 1017–1025.

[12] Abdel-Rahman, S. M., Reed, M. D., Wells, T. G., Kearns, G. L. (2007): *Considerations in the rational design and conduct of phase I/II pediatric clinical trials: avoiding the problems and pitfalls*, in: Clinical Pharmacology & Therapeutics 81 (4), 483–494; Kauffman, R. E. (2000): *Clinical trials in children: problems and pitfalls*, in: Paediatric Drugs 2 (6), 411–418.

[13] See Table 1.

[14] International Conference of Harmonization of Technical Requirements for Registration of Pharmaceuticals for Human Use (2000): *Clinical Investigation of Medicinal Products in the Paediatric Population. E11*. URL http://www.ich.org/fileadmin/Public_Web_Site/ICH_Products/Guidelines/Efficacy/E11/Step4/E11_Guideline.pdf [28 August 2017]; International Conference of Harmonization of Technical Requirements for Registration of Pharmaceuticals for Human Use (2016): *E11(R1) Addendum: Clinical Investigation of Medicinal Products in the Pediatric Population. Concept Paper. Step 2b Presentation and Work Plan. Draft Guideline*.

Differences in Legal Age for Informed Consents

In most of the European countries, 18 years is the legal age also for the independent Informed Consent (IC) for participating CTs, but with the following exceptions: 14 years in Austria, 15 years in Finland, Denmark and the Netherlands, and 16 years the UK. These exceptions come with certain limitations and with obligation to notify parents or legal guardians. However, across all the European countries, thirty-two different age groupings for recommended additional assent or consent needed from the child participating in the CT. Only three countries (Croatia, Lithuania and Slovakia) have not specified age groups for assent or consent.[15] According to the new CTR, *"Minor, means a subject who is, according to the law of Member States concerned, under the age of legal competence to give informed consent"* (Chapter I, Article 2, Recital 18).[16] By this definition, the "legal competent age", can remain lower (such as 15 years in Finland) for the independent consent with some national more detailed requirements (e.g. notification for the legal representatives).

Differences in Legal Signatures

Due to these national legal variations, there are differences also in the requirements of signatures from parents or legal representatives. The majority of the European countries (63%) require the signatures of both parents in addition to the child's own assent or consent.[17] In the new CTR, the term "*Legally designated representative*" is defined in the singular form (Chapter I, Article 2, Recital 20). Moreover, later in the CTR text, the first condition for the minor's participation in CT is that "*the informed consent of their legally designated representative has been obtained*" (Chapter 5, Article 32, Recital 1.a) – also in singular form.[18] Reflected by these regulative conditions, it could be anticipated that the widely used current practice of two signatures (of both parents) could change in several European countries after the CTR implementation.

Differences in Terminology

The terms "consent" and "assent" are not uniformly defined in general guidelines, nor in the European legal texts. Moreover, these are not harmonized across

---

[15] European Network of Paediatric Research at the European Medicines Agency 2017; Lepola et al. 2016.
[16] European Commission 2014.
[17] European Network of Paediatric Research at the European Medicines Agency 2017; Lepola et al. 2016.
[18] European Commission 2014.

Europe nor internationally. Some European countries, like Finland, use the term "consent" for both minors (older children below legal adult age) and parents (legal representatives).[19] Generally, the term "assent" refers to a child's or minor's non-legal agreement (not valid on its own), and an additional parental (legal representative) signature (consent) is always required before the participation of the child in a CT is legally accepted. The term "consent" refers to the legal signature(s) by the parents (legal representatives) or by a minor when he/she has reached the legal age of adulthood for participating in CT independently. The new CTR uses both terms; "*assent*" generally when referring to the minor's own opinion prior the participation decisions, and "*consent*" as a legal agreement.[20]

Pediatric Consents for Biological Samples and Biobanks

Biomedical research and CTs are increasingly exploring the impact of human genes and environment, in addition to the etiology of the diseases, by combining these information sources in order to develop new and more specific medications, also for pediatric conditions and especially for rare diseases occurring in early childhood. The development of biobanks, collecting the genetic information via biological samples, occurs in all European countries, but in different timelines. The regulative texts around biobanks seem to follow the same pattern as for CTs; some countries have established forward-looking national laws for biobanks covering children and adolescents,[21] while broader discussion about consents, sample research findings and age ranges has just started, and have not yet reached consensus among professionals. As these practices and the regulative framework will differ between countries, it further complicates the challenges for CTs.[22]

---

[19] European Network of Paediatric Research at the European Medicines Agency 2017; Lepola et al. 2016.
[20] European Commission 2014.
[21] Soini, S. (2013): *Finland on a road towards a modern legal biobanking infrastructure*, in: European Journal of Health Law 20 (3), 289–94.
[22] Kaye, J., Briceño Moraia, L., Curren, L., Bell, J., Mitchell, C., Soini, S., Hoppe, N., Øien, M., Rial-Sebbag, E. (2016): *Consent for Biobanking: The Legal Frameworks of Countries in the BioSHaRE-EU Project*, in: Biopreservation and Biobanking 14 (3), 195–200; Kranendonk, E. J., Ploem, M. C., Hennekam, R. C. M. (2016): *Regulating biobanking with children's tissue: a legal analysis and the experts' view*, in: European Journal of Human Genetics 24 (1), 30–36; Kranendonk, E. J., Hennekam, R. C., Ploem, M. C. (2017): *Paediatric biobanking: Dutch experts reflecting on appropriate legal standards for practice*, in: European Journal of Pediatrics 176 (1), 75–82.

Social Complexity Challenge All Stakeholders

Demanding Rehearsal for Sponsors and Regulators

During the ten years of Pediatric Regulation,[23] all stakeholders have had an opportunity to practice how the pediatric CTs should be designed, processed, evaluated, assessed and conducted; in the spirit of the regulation.[24] It has not been easy rehearsal, as it correlates with the numbers of new PIPs submitted by the pharmaceutical companies, but also in the numbers of actually started new Pediatric CTs, registered into the European Clinical Trials Registry.[25] Generally, the annual number of pediatric CTs has been on average 400, representing approx. 10% proportion of all CTs (on average 4000) registered into the Eudra-CT since 2006. The PIP is mandatory to design for all (adult) products, when applying Marketing Authorization in European markets, if the PDCO have not agreed on the waiver (no need to study in pediatric population). One PIP may include the requirement to conduct several pediatric CTs at different phases (e.g. non-clinical, Phases I-III).

In November 2016, the European Commission launched a public consultation for its second report on the Paediatric Regulation after nearly ten years of implementation. The EMA/PDCO prepared a 10-year-report for the consultation based on experience with implementing the Regulation.[26] The report shows that pediatric medicine development has improved in the European medicines regulatory network over the last ten years, but also highlights the challenges to be addressed. In this report, the number of agreed PIPs was 860, but the completed PIPs by the Pharma companies was only 100 (12%). This was seen also in a number of new registered pediatric CTs (in a CT at least 1 recruited participant has been under 18-years of age), as the number was increased only 2% (from 9.3% to 11.5%) from 2006. The final EU Commission 10-year-report was published in October 2017.[27]

Lack of Material and Uniformity

All stakeholders know that this slow development is mainly due to the nature of Pediatric Regulation (i.e. product development focused primarily to adult conditions), but also due to the deficiency on several sectors; experience, uniform

---

[23] European Commission 2006.
[24] European Medicines Agency (2012): *Policy on the determination of the condition(s) for a Paediatric Investigation Plan/Waiver (scope of the PIP/waiver)*. URL http://www.ema.europa.eu/docs/en_GB/document_library/Other/2012/09/WC500133065.pdf [31 August 2017].
[25] European Medicines Agency (2017): *European clinical trial database. EudraCT statistics*. URL https://eudract.ema.europa.eu/statistics.html [31 August 2017].
[26] European Medicines Agency 2016.
[27] Lepola et al. 2016.

guidance, specific training and harmonized and specifically designed materials for pediatric CTs. Therefore, especially ECs repeatedly receive incomplete documentation, not aimed for pediatric CTs. The IC or assent documents have been too complex to understand, and too extent to read and comprehend. Furthermore, every Pharma Company and Contract Research Organization (CRO) has their own documentation templates in addition to their own guidelines for designing these documents. In European level multicenter pediatric CTs, this phenomenon exists in a form of hundreds of different document templates submitted to ECs. Moreover, the heterogeneity of ECs composition, different timelines and great legislative variability between countries, constitutes extra complications causing unnecessary work, repeated amendments, re-evaluations and finally – the loss of time and money.[28]

Lack of Knowledge and Experience in Practice

There are specific challenges associated also with the pediatric patient recruitment. In case of acute illness, rare disease or in emergency medical care situations, the circumstances may prevent normal recruitment and communication for understanding given information, bringing along difficulties of recruiting in timely manner. Partly due to these facts, the recruiting systems and methods without justifications for pediatric patients has caused extra work for the industry and ECs when assessing the suitability of the adult recruitment methods for pediatric CTs. The recruitment arrangements require specific considerations.[29]

During the past ten years, the clinical personnel of the various clinical research networks, including investigators and experts and research nurses, faced new demands when the number of CT proposals in the early PIP development phase (i.e.

---

[28] Hernandez, R., Cooney, M., Dualé, C., Gálvez, M., Gaynor, S., Kardos, G., Kubiak, C., Mihaylov, S., Pleiner, J., Ruberto, G., Sanz, N., Skoog, M., Souri, P., Stiller, C. O., Strenge-Hesse, A., Vas, A., Winter, D., Carné, X. (2009): *Harmonisation of ethics committees' practice in 10 European countries*, in: Journal of Medical Ethics 35 (11), 696–700; Altavilla, A., Manfredi, C., Baiardi, P., Dehlinger-Kremer, M., Galletti, P., Pozuelo, A. A., Chaplin, J., Ceci, A. (2012*): Impact of the new european paediatric regulatory framework on ethics committees: overview and perspectives*, in: Acta Paediatrica 101 (1), e27–32; De Feo, G., Chiabrando, G., Cannovo, N., Galluccio, A., Tomino, C. (2012): *Harmonization of the practice of independent ethics committees in Italy: project E-submission*, in: PLOS One 7 (11), e48906; Gülmez, S. E., Lignot-Maleyran, S., de Vries, C. S., Sturkenboom, M., Micon, S., Hamoud, F., Blin, P., Moore, N. (2012): *Administrative complexities for a European observational study despite directives harmonising requirements*, in: Pharmacoepidemiology and Drug Safety 21 (8), 851–856; Veerus, P., Lexchin, J., Hemminki, E. (2014): *Legislative regulation and ethical governance of medical research in different European Union countries*, in: Journal of Medical Ethics 40 (6), 409–413.

[29] Stocks, J., Lum, S. (2016): *Back to school: challenges and rewards of engaging young children in scientific research*, in: Archives of Disease in Childhood 101 (9), 785–787.

feasibility questionnaires) have increased across Europe. With these proposals, Pharma Companies and CRO's search for prospects for PIP development and possible CT sites (hospitals, clinics) and research personnel for the CT conduction. As other stakeholder groups, the majority of the pediatric research personnel has very short history and experience of pediatric CTs and the knowledge of the research on new medicines in his population. Indeed, there are relatively very few pediatric experts across the stakeholders.[30] In general, to date, there have been very limited options of comprehensive training programs or short courses for clinical personnel, especially in non-English speaking countries. Only recently, the EU-funded framework programs have provided proper training programs for all stakeholders around pediatric medicines and CTs.[31]

Lack of Public Awareness

Immediately following the historically low research activity of pediatric CTs, these have not been part of the daily routines of normal medical care for large populations. Therefore, pediatric CTs are not commonly well known by the public. During the past few years, the awareness of the public increased due to active campaigns by patient organizations partly funded by EU framework programs. Only recently, the authorities and several learned societies have started to notice the importance of the voice of pediatric patients and their families.[32] The opinions and experiences of patients and parents have become very important part in the development process of new medicinal products; from drug discovery to CTs in practice.[33] As a result, since 2006 (The Children Specialty's Young Person's Advisory Group, UK) new Young Person's Advisory Groups (YPAG) have been established in to several countries in Europe. Now, YPAGs collaborate internationally, taking the more active role as partners on various pediatric research.[34]

---

[30] Hoppu, K. (2008): *Paediatric clinical pharmacology: at the beginning of a new era*, in: European Journal of Clinical Pharmacology 64 (2), 201–205.

[31] Turner, M. A., Catapano, M., Hirschfeld, S., Giaquinto, C. (2014): *Global Research in Paediatrics. Paediatric drug development: the impact of evolving regulations*, in: Advanced Drug Delivery Reviews 73, 2–13.

[32] European Commission (2017): *RESPECT: Relating Expectations and Needs to the Participation and Empowerment of Children in Clinical Trials. Project overview*. URL http://www.patientneeds.eu/RESPECT.html [29 August 2017].

[33] Tume L. N., Preston J., Blackwood B. (2016): *Parents' and young people's involvement in designing a trial of ventilator weaning*, in: Nursing in Critical Care 21 (3), e10–18.

[34] International Children's Advisory Network (2017): *eYPAgnet-iCAN Research*. URL https://www.icanresearch.org/chapters/eypagnet/ [29 August 2017].

New Era for Ethics Committees

There are still more than 1000 EC's in Europe, which results in the substantial variability of EC compositions and practices, with consequently a certain degree of inconsistency as the data requirements change between ECs and can vary greatly.[35] Due to the huge amount of EC's, it is not possible to maintain a relationship with all of them and as they are also all different and independent, and the practice for one EC will not necessarily work for the other. As this setting has been challenging for adult CTs it may be expected to have additional challenges when the number of pediatric CTs increases in Europe. Furthermore, some extra challenges are expected when the ECs faces major changes due to new CTR implementation. It will remain to be seen how the ECs will be nationally organized and how the CTR's strict timeline affects to EC operations across Europe.

Tackle the Challenges by European Level Collaboration

The European Network for Pediatric Research – Enpr-EMA

The objective of the Paediatric Regulation (Regulation EC No 1901/20061) is to foster high-quality ethical research in order to increase the availability of safe and effective medicinal products authorised for use in the paediatric population. To meet this objective, the European Medicines Agency (EMA) established Enpr-EMA, The European Network of Paediatric Research at the European Medicines Agency, in March 2011.[36] Enpr-EMA is a network of pediatric research networks (national, age specific, disease specific, therapeutic area and knowledge specific), investigators and centres. These networks are Enpr-EMA's members and are required to fulfil certain criteria for the membership. The operational centre of Enpr-EMA is the Coordinating Group (CG), which is responsible for the network's long- and short-term strategy. The EMA provides the secretariat support to various Enpr-EMA activities, such as meetings, ensuring the exchange of information between the network partners and stakeholders. Enpr-EMA works by allowing networking and collaboration with members from within and outside the EU, including academia and the pharmaceutical industry.

---

[35] Altavilla et al. 2012; Hernandez et al. 2009; Veerus, Lexchin, Hemminki 2014; De Feo et al. 2012; Gülmez et al. 2012.

[36] European Medicines Agency (2017): European Network of Paediatric Research at the European Medicines Agency (Enpr-EMA). URL http://www.ema.europa.eu/ema/index.jsp?curl=pages/partners_and_networks/general/general_content_000303.jsp&mid=WC0b01ac05801df74a [31 August 2017]; Ruperto, N., Eichler, I., Herold, R., Vassal, G., Giaquinto, C., Hjorth, L., Valls-i-Soler, A., Peters, C., Helms, P. J., Raymond, A. S. (2012): *A European network of paediatric research at the European Medicines Agency (Enpr-EMA)*, in: Archives of Disease in Childhood 97, 185–188.

Enpr-EMA Mandate for Several Working Groups

One of the practical aims of Enpr-EMA is to find solutions to emerge need (e.g. challenges) related to the pediatric CTs and the development of medicines for children. For this purpose, Enpr-EMA mandated to form several ad hoc Working Groups (WG) among the members in 2013. These WGs were tasked with several objectives to make the most of Enpr-EMA pediatric research networks by: 1) facilitating communication between the stakeholders involved in pediatric CTs, 2) gathering examples of good practice and 3) developing pragmatic proposals for these examples and new ideas, implementable within approximately six months. Afterwards these ideas will be disseminated across Enpr-EMA members and across the stakeholders groups.

Enpr-EMA Ethics Working Group (WG4)

The Enpr-EMA Working Group 4 (WG4) focuses particularly on these ethical issues, and operates under the title *"Dialogue and Interaction with Ethics Committees"*. The WG4 consists of ten experts and professionals representing academia, Pharma Companies and CROs, and specified to work in the area of pediatric CTs.

The "Tool Kit" – a Table of European Requirements for IC and Assents

The first deliverable of the WG4 was a "Tool Kit" – *Informed Consent and Assent for Paediatric Clinical Trials in Europe*. This "Tool Kit" is a table including 27 national IC and assent requirements listed by individual country (25 European Union Member States and 2 European Free Trade Association countries) and it was published on Enpr-EMA website on 18 December 2015.[37] The Enpr-EMA Secretariat updated the "Tool Kit" until today (2017). This Tool Kit being publicly available free of costs on the Enpr-EMA website meets the main aim set to WGs. The related article was published on 25 May 2016.[38]

Response to Public Consultation of the "Paediatric Ethics Guideline"

One of the central ethical guidelines supporting for pediatric clinical trials in Europe has been the "Ethical Considerations for Clinical Trials on Medicinal

---

[37] European Network of Paediatric Research at the European Medicines Agency 2017.
[38] Lepola 2016.

Products Conducted with Minors" ("*Paediatric Ethics Guideline*") originally published by EU Commission's Ad Hoc group in 2008.[39] Second actual deliverable of the WG4 was a response to this "Paediatric Ethics Guideline". The consultation represented the response from Enpr-EMA, its working groups and partners and was contributed by the European Forum for Good Clinical Practice, Children's Medicines Working Party (EFGCP CMWP) in collaboration with a small group of EMA PDCO members. The consultation document was submitted on 30 August 2016.[40] The revision of the "Pediatric Ethics Guideline" was published in September 2017.[41]

"IC / Assent Template Guidance Document" for Paediatric CTs

The third deliverable of the WG4 is about *"Informed Consent / Assent template Guidance Document for paediatric CTs"*, and has been prepared during the year 2016–2017. The document template has been reviewed by three European YPAGs: The KIDS Barcelona (Spanish YPAG of Hospital San Joan De Deu), the Generation R (National Young Persons' Advisory Group made up of local groups across the UK) Liverpool's Team and the ScotCRN (Scottish Children's Research Network). These groups commented the usefulness and text contents. The Guidance Document will be finalized after the careful review against the new *"Pediatric Ethics Guideline"* together with the comments of the experts from the European Academy of Pediatrics (EAP). The document is based on the identification of required elements for the ICs and assents. The Guidance Document will be made publicly available on Enpr-EMA website.

---

[39] European Commission (2008): *Ethical Considerations for Clinical Trials on Medicinal Products with the Paediatric Population. Recommendations of the Ad hoc group for the development of implementing guidelines for Directive 2001/20/EC relating to good clinical practice in the conduct of clinical trials on medicinal products for human use.* URL https://ec.europa.eu/health/sites/health/files/files/eudralex/vol-10/ethical_considerations_en.pdf [31 August 2017].

[40] European network of paediatric research at the European Medicines Academy (2016): *Consultation on the revision of "Ethical Considerations for Clinical Trials on Medicinal products conducted with Minors": a response from Enpr-EMA and partners.* URL https://ec.europa.eu/health/sites/health/files/files/clinicaltrials/2016_06_pc_guidelines/gl_1_resp_enpr_ema.pdf [28 August 2017].

[41] Nordicpedmed. URL www.nordicpedmed.com [15 January 2018]; Korppi, M., Lepola, P., Vettenranta, K., Pakkala, S., Hoppu, K. (2013): *Limited impact of EU paediatric regulation on Finnish clinical trials highlights need for Nordic collaboration.* Acta Paediatrica 102 (11), 1035–1040.

The Nordic Network for Pediatric Medicines – NORDICPEDMED

The Nordic investigators network for Pediatric Medicines (NordicPedMed) is a collaborative Nordic network, aiming to improve the health care of children and adolescents by enhancing Nordic research collaboration. NordicPedMed simultaneously supports the development of national research networks of centers (hospitals) and investigators in all five Nordic countries (Denmark, Finland, Iceland, Norway, and Sweden), and the establishment of a Nordic-level network for pediatric CTs of medicinal products and other therapies. NordicPedMed was initiated in 2014-2016, with funding from the Nordic Council of Ministers and NordForsk, through a 3-year NordicTrial Alliance (NTA) project, and it was official launched on 1st June 2017. The development continues during the following years.[42]

The Pediatric Clinical Research Infrastructure Network – PedCRIN

The Paediatric Clinical Research Infrastructure Network (PedCRIN) brings together the European Clinical Research Infrastructure Network (ECRIN) and the founding partners of the European Paediatric Clinical Trial Research Infrastructure (EPCT-RI) to develop capacity for the management of multinational, non-commercial, pediatric CTs. PedCRIN is a four-year project funded by the EU's Horizon 2020 program, launched on 1st January 2017.

PedCRIN will effectively bridge pediatricians and other partners across Europe (and internationally) to combine resources and expertise to conduct and manage robust studies, while minimizing risk and protecting the child participants. The aim of PedCRIN is to develop the necessary tools and capacity to enhance the quality, safety, efficacy and ethical standards of multinational academic pediatric CTs. In addition, YPAGs and families have the essential role in the PedCRIN project across the work packages.[43]

Ideas to Improve Ethics for Pediatric CTs on Practical Level

Example of National Research Network – FinPedMed

FinPedMed (Finnish Investigators Network for Pediatric Medicines), established in 2007, is a non-juridical joint venture of all (5) Finnish university hospitals operating on an open, non-profit service concept basis to promote both academic

---

[42] Nordicpedmed. URL www.nordicpedmed.com [15 January 2018]; Korppi, M., Lepola, P., Vettenranta, K., Pakkala, S., Hoppu, K. (2013): *Limited impact of EU paediatric regulation on Finnish clinical trials highlights need for Nordic collaboration.* Acta Paediatrica 102 (11), 1035–1040.

[43] PedCRIN. URL www.ecrin.org/activities/pedcrin [28 August 2017].

and sponsored research in Finland. FinPedMed, a Finnish national network and a member of the Enpr-EMA, has developed various materials and a tailored training program to support the high ethical aspects of the paediatric CTs. Materials are designed for investigators, and in addition to companies designing and conducting the paediatric CTs.[44]

FinPedMed Picture Cards

During the year 2008, a group of experts stated that the use of illustrative material to aid the understanding patient information has thus far been minimal, and created a set of picture cards for investigators to help pediatric trial participants understand the content of patient information. The planning of the cards based on the knowledge of both developmental and educational psychology, as well as neuropsychology. The content for the pictures was collected by various methods. Children (between 1 and 6 years) in a Day Care Centre commented anonymously on the pictures, and these were modified to be better suitable for the objects and situations in question based on these comments. FinPedMed Picture Cards exist in printed form inside a folder, including a set of 31 pictures of both objects and situations. All Picture Cards include labels in Finnish, Swedish and English. Picture Cards are usable widely by all professionals in clinical work.[45]

FinPedMed IC Templates for All Age Groups

In 2009, a group of experts designed IC documents and trial information sheets for children (under the age of 18) for all age groups and their guardians to be used in CTs. All document templates are accepted by all EC's in Finland and are available in Finnish, Swedish and in English. These document templates take into account the child's developmental stage and level of understanding, the guardians' need for information and the laws regulating trials in Finland and Europe. The document templates are intended for the use of investigators and the Pharma companies conducting CTs in Finland. The uniform documents will improve the ethical quality of trials as well as speed up the time it takes for the EC approvals at a national level.[46]

---

[44] Finpedmed. URL www.finpedmed.com [28 August 2017].
[45] Finpedmed (2017): *Picture Cards for paediatric clinical trials*. URL http://www.finpedmed.fi/index.php?page=1152&lang=2 [28 August 2017].
[46] Finpedmed (2017): *Document templates, web-sites and guidelines for pediatric clinical trials*. URL http://www.finpedmed.fi/index.php?page=500&lang=2 [28 August 2017].

FinPedMed Tailored Research Nurse Training Program

For each new trial, the investigator needs a trained study nurse with research experience and knowledge. Lack of knowledge causes limited communication about CTs, which in turn lowers the interest to take part in CTs among patients and families. For this reason, FinPedMed developed specifically tailored and locally adapted a Paediatric Research Training Program of four (4) Credit Units. The curriculum has been designed by FinPedMed Executive Board together with the clinical research units and pediatric clinics and it covers many important subjects around medical ethics; legal, regulatory, pharmacological, operational and pure practical issues. The program includes lectures according to the hospital's own processes, with the content focused on pediatric nurses. The training program started as a pilot project in Tampere University Hospital (2015-2016) and since that in two other University Hospitals during 2016-2017. To date 30 newly trained pediatric research nurses have completed the training program together with Good Clinical Practice (GCP) test.

Future Trends & Prospects for Paediatric Clinical Research

Electronic Applications and E-documentation

Children and adolescents are currently better known as; "digital generation". The use of social media in various forms, all types of e-services and e-documentation are the most natural part of their life. The trend of future CTs is also developing around e-services in all formats, leading to the increased need for new CT design, e-Privacy rules and new prospects for harmonized procedures and collaboration with all stakeholders.

For this development, we will need to seek advice from the children and young people, as experts, to develop the most feasible patient information, ICs or assents and other trial documentation, to ensure high quality and secure medical research environment. In addition, the future trends and prospects will include electronically supported trial documentation and (partly) remote trial conduction. This speeds up the development of new guidance, legislation and research programs across all stakeholders, together with companies specialized in electronic data and documentation. YPAGs present the best consultants of the user-friendly and feasible digital e-applications of interactive multimedia, as well as e-ICs and e-assents.[47]

---

[47] Pfizer (2011): *Pfizer Conducts First "Virtual" Clinical Trial Allowing Patients to Participate Regardless Of Geography. Pilot Study Will Compare Results to Previous Trial Data to Assess Validity of New Approach.* URL http://press.pfizer.com/press-release/pfizer-conducts-first-virtual-clinical-trial-allowing-patients-participate-regardless- [28 August 2017]; Tait, A. R.,

Conclusion

The current wide variation in documentation and guidance presents obstacles for multinational pediatric clinical research and CTs in Europe. Solving these, would need more uniform, commonly accepted standards and guidance together with clear definitions and common requirements, leading to harmonized processes.

Those designing and reviewing pediatric CTs should have appropriate expertise. Consultations for the pediatric clinical research should be done by using the opinions and advice of the real experts of the specific field of pediatrics. Those conducting research involving minors should have appropriate expertise in form of official professional certificates. Children and their families should be involved in research from inception, in its design and the material to be used. Awareness and good communication, as well as openness and transparency, are important parts of high ethical standards and behind the success of modern pediatric CTs.

To find solutions to all of these challenges, we need training, clinical experience, and changes in practice with support from regulators. More good practices and new ideas need to be shared among research networks and other stakeholders. In addition, we need European level training programs and increased communication methods, and more personnel, resources and funding.

The development is only through changes in attitudes and changes in working methods with common interest in more open manners. Clinical research networks, industry and authorities together with learned societies and patient groups are all substantially capable of improving the pediatric clinical research in practice. All European stakeholders must address the need and build more on networking, by creating new collaborative methods in order to tackle these issues together.

Voepel-Lewis, T., Levine, R. (2015): *Using digital multimedia to improve parents' and children's understanding of clinical trials*, in: Archives of Disease in Childhood 100 (6), 589–593; Tait, A.R., Voepel-Lewis, T. (2015): *Digital multimedia: a new approach for informed consent?*, in: The Journal of the American Medical Association 313 (5), 463–464.

Table 1. Table of Current Global Informed Consent or Assent Age Definitions for Minors for Clinical Research in Literature and Legal Frame *(not published previously).*

Organization / Institution – Convention / Declaration / Guideline / Law (enty into force, year)	Age Definitions of a Child	Age Frame Definitions of Competency / Capacity (understanding and make judgements in health care) for ASSENT or CONSENT Mentioned in the Document	Guideline Definitions for Age Groups or Age Limits for ASSENT or CONSENT
UNICEF – Convention on the Rights of Child (1990)[48]	Under 18 years.	Not defined.	
CIOMS – International Ethical Guideline for Biomedical Research Involving Human Subjects (2002)[49]	Not mentioned. Endorce all general ethical principles, and international human rights instruments.	Children over 12 or 13 years.	– 0-11 years; no recommendations. – Own assent from children since 12 or 13 years of age. Otherwise refers to general age of adulthood 18 years according to the UNESCO, YK, WHO, UNICEF, and WMA.
UN – Universal Declaration of Human Rights (1948)[50]	"A full age", "childhood" and "child" mentioned. Not defined.	Not defined.	
Belmont Report – U.S. Department of Health & Human Services (1978)[51]	"Children", "infant" and "young children" mentioned. Not defined.	Not defined.	

---

[48] United Nations 1990.
[49] The Council for International Organizations of Medical Sciences (CIOMS) in collaboration with the World Health Organization (WHO) (2002): *International Ethical Guideline for Biomedical Research Involving Human Subjects*. URL https://cioms.ch/shop/product/international-ethical-guidelines-for-biomedical-research-involving-human-subjects-2 [29 August 2017].
[50] United Nations (1948): *The Universal Declaration of Human Rights*. URL http://www.un.org/en/documents/udhr/ [29 August 2017].
[51] National Commission for the Protection of Human Subjects of Biomedical and Behavioral Research (1978): *The Belmont Report: Ethical Principles and Guidelines for the Commission for the Protection of Human Subjects of Biomedical and Behavioral Research*. URL https://repository.library.georgetown.edu/handle/10822/779133 [29August2017].

WHO – Guidelines for good clinical practice (GCP) for trials on pharmaceutical products (1995)[52]	"A voulnerable group", "incapable research subject" and "child" mentioned. Not defined.[5]	Not defined.	
WMA – Declaration of Helsinki (2013)[53]	"A voulnerable group" and "incapable research subject" mentioned. Not defined.	Not defined.	
Council of Europe – ETS no. 164 – Convention for the Protection of Human Rights and Dignity of the Human Being with regard to the Application of Biology and Medicine: Convention on Human Rights and Biomedicine (1997)[54]	"A minor by law" and "person not able to consent" mentioned. Refers to national legislation.	Not defined.	
UNESCO – Universal Declaration on Bioethics and Human Rights (2005)[55]	"A person without capacity to consent" mentioned. Refers to domestic law.	Not defined.	

---

[52] World Health Organization (1995): *WHO Guidelines for good clinical practice (GCP) for trials on pharmaceutical products*, in: Technical Report Series, No. 850, 1995, Annex 3. URL http://apps.who.int/medicinedocs/pdf/whozip13e/whozip13e.pdf [15 March 2018].

[53] World Medical Association (2013): *WMA Declaration of Helsinki – Ethical Principles for Medical Research Involving Human Subjects*. 64th WMA General Assembly, Fortaleza, Brazil, October 2013. URL https://www.wma.net/publications/wma-doh-1964-2014/ (Availability only by orders to WMA) [16 January 2018].

[54] Council of Europe (1999): *Convention for the Protection of Human Rights and Dignity of the Human Being with regard to the Application of Biology and Medicine: Convention on Human Rights and Biomedicine*. URL http://conventions.coe.int/Treaty/en/Treaties/Html/164.htm [29 August 2017].

[55] United Nations Educational, Scientific and Cultural Organization (2005): *UNESCO Universal Declaration on Bioethics and Human Rights*. URL http://www.unesco.org/new/en/social-and-human-sciences/themes/bioethics/bioethics-and-human-rights/ [29 August 2017].

AAP – Guidelines for the Ethical Conduct of Studies to Evaluate Drugs in Pediatric Population (2010)[56] – refers to Federal Regulations listed in Ethical Conduct of Clinical Research Involving Children (National Institute of Medicine, 2004)[57]	[9]"Children, adolescents, and young adults"; age more precisely defined by local laws (state law or federal statute, state limits between 16 and 21 years). Includes special definitions for "emancipated and mature minors" under legal age, but considered as an adult e.g. for clinical research. [10]Age of Majority varies between 18 and 21, emancipated conditions, mature minor status and minor consent age for certain conditions / disorders varies between the States.	[9]Recommendations: Intellectual age of 7 yrs and above – active agreement participation, developmentally normal children between 8 and 14 yrs – assent genrally acceptable, adolescents between 12 and 18 (dependent on region) – assent process as an adult IC process.	0-6 years: no recommendations. Assent – child's own assent since 7 years. Can be waived / not mandatory, if the child cannot give assent in person (due to medical condition or other reason). Assent – Own assent by adolescent since 12 years until reaching the legal adulthood. Consent – Emancipated minors due to marriage, parenthood or other reason, can give their own consent and consent on behalf of their own child / children.
U.S. – 21 CFR (FDA Regulations); 50, 201, 814[58]	Labeling regulations for drugs/ biologics: 0 to <17 years [21 CFR 201.57(c)(9)(iv)] Pediatric Medical Device Safety Improvement Act: 0 to 21 years [Section 814.3(2)(s)], Additional Protections for Children (subpart D):" Persons who have not attained the legal age for consent to treatments or procedures involved in clinical investigations, under the applicable law of the jurisdiction in which the clinical investigation will be conducted" [21 CFR 50.3(o)].	Not defined.	

---

[56] Shaddy, R. E., Denne S. C., the Committee on Drugs and Committee on Pediatric Research of the American Academy of Pediatrics (2010): *Guidelines for the Ethical Conduct of Studies to Evaluate Drugs in Pediatric Populations*, in: Pediatrics 125 (4), 850–860.

[57] Field, M. J., Behrman, R. E., Institute of Medicine (US) Committee on Clinical Research Involving Children (eds.) (2004): *Ethical Conduct of Clinical Research Involving Children*, Washington (DC). URL http://www.ncbi.nlm.nih.gov/books/NBK25557/ [29 August 2017].

[58] U.S. Department of Health and Human Services, U.S. Food and Drug Administration (2017): *CFR – Code of Federal Regulations, Title 21*; Parts 50, 201 and 814. URL 50: http://www.accessdata.fda.gov/scripts/cdrh/cfdocs/cfcfr/CFRSearch.cfm?CFRPart=50, 201: http://www.accessdata.fda.gov/scripts/cdrh/cfdocs/cfCFR/CFRSearch.cfm?CFRPart=201, 814: http://www.acce

EAP – Informed consent/assent in children (2003)[59], Ethical principles and operational guidelines for good clinical practice in paediatric research (2004)[60] and Guidelines for informed consent in biomedical research involving paediatric populations as research participants (2003)[61]	[12]Refers to UN Convention[1], and generally EU laws; the age of majority is 18 yrs.[13] Includes 7 age groups for pediatric population; 0-16/18 yrs.	[12]Based on literature; the ability to understand can be earliest from 9 yrs and above.[14] The guideline principle 8; definition of a child should reflect the legal age definitions of the country of the reserch (national law).	– no age-specific guidance – recommended to ask child's own Assent as soon as child is able to read and write Includes 7 different aggroupings for children between 0-16/18 years; (below 28 weeks, below 36 weeks, 0-27 days, 28 days-23 months, 2-5 years., 6-11 years., 12-16/18 years). – Refers generally to the declations of the United Nations and European legislation, when the legal age of adulthood is generally 18 years.
ICH – Guideline for Good Clinical Practice E6(R1) (1996)[62] *Addendum E6(R2) adopted in Europe by CHMP, 15 December 2016, issued as EMA/CHMP/ICH/135/1995*	"Vulnerable Subjects", including minors (1.61), "subjects who can only be enrolled in the trial with the consent of the subject's legally acceptable representative, e.g. minors" (4.8.12)	Not defined.	

ssdata.fda.gov/scripts/cdrh/cfdocs/cfcfr/CFRSearch.cfm?CFRPart=814 [29 August 2017].

[59] De Lourdes Levy, M., Larcher, V., Kurz, R., Ethics Working Group of the Confederation of European Specialists in Paediatrics (CESP) (2003): *Informed consent/assent in children. Statement of the Ethics Working Group of the Confederation of European Specialists in Paediatrics (CESP)*, in: European Journal of Pediatrics 162 (9), 629–633.

[60] Gill, D., Ethics Working Group of the Confederation of European Specialists in Paediatrics (2004):*Ethical principles and operational guidelines for good clinical practice in paediatric research. Recommendations of the Ethics Working Group of the Confederation of European Specialists in Paediatrics (CESP)*, in: European Journal of Pediatrics 163 (2), 53–57.

[61] Gill, D., Ethics Working Group of the Confederation of European Specialists in Pediatrics (2003): *Guidelines for informed consent in biomedical research involving paediatric populations as research participants*, in: European Journal of Pediatrics 162 (7-8), 455–458.

[62] International Conference of Harmonization (1996): *ICH Guideline for good Clinical Practice E6(R2)*. URL http://www.ich.org/products/guidelines/efficacy/article/efficacy-guidelines.html Addendum E6(R2) has been implemented in Europe, Adopted by CHMP, 15 December 2016, issued as EMA/CHMP/ICH/135/1995 [29 August 2017].

ICH E 11 – Clinical Investigation of Medicinal Products in the Paediatric Population (2000)[63] Revised (R1) Addendum published in April 2018. (see the correspondent text reference)	"A pediatric patient" and "Pediatric population" mentioned; includes example categorization; preterm newborn infants, term newborn infants (0 to 27 days), infants and toddlers (28 days to 23 months), children (2 to 11 years), and adolescents (12 to 16-18 years (dependent on region)). Addendum includes age classification specifications.	Not defined. 2.6.3.: "As a rule, a pediatric subject is legally unable to provide informed consent." "Fully informed consent should be obtained from the legal guardian in accordance with regional laws or regulations." "Participants should assent to enroll in a study (age of assent to be determined by IRB's/IEC's or be consistent with local legal requirements). Participants of appropriate intellectual maturity should personally sign and date either a separately designed, written assent form or the written informed consent."	– no recommendations for consents. Addendum includes glossary consent / assent definitions.
EU Commission – EU Clinical Trials Directive (2001)[64]	"Children" and "vulnerable population" (3), "Minors" Article 4.	Not defined. "The informed consent of the parents or legal representative; consent must represent the minor's presumed will and may be revoked at any time, without detriment to the minor, and the minor has received information according to its capacity of understanding."	

---

[63] International Conference of Harmonization (2000): *ICH E11(R1) – Clinical Investigation of Medicinal Products in the Paediatric Population*. URL http://www.ich.org/products/guidelines/efficacy/article/efficacy-guidelines.html [29 August 2017].

[64] EU Commission (2011): *Directive 2001/20/EC of the European Parliament and of the Council of 4 April 2001 on the approximation of the laws, regulations and administrative provisions of the Member Status relating to the implementation of good clinical practice in the conduct of clinical trials on medicinal products for human use*, in: Official Journal of the European Union, L 121/34–44. URL http://ec.europa.eu/health/human-use/clinical-trials/directive/index_en.htm [29 August 2017].

RCPCH – Royal College of Pediatrics and Child Health Ethics Advisory Committee, U.K. (2014)[65] Guidance on clinical research and Guidelines for pediatric medical research (2000)[66] UK-MRC – UK Medical Research Council (2004)[67]	[18] Refers to U.K. Clinical Trial Regulation "A minor is a child less than 16 yrs" and [19] refers U.K. law; "A child is under 18 yrs old".	By law; 16 yrs or older is able to give independent consent. RCPCH view; children over 7 yrs are able to give assent, and children over 12-14 yrs may have near adult capacity.	[20]Refers to national medical research act, where the minor is under 16 years, but in other cases, the minor is under 18 years. If the child's parents are themselves under 16 years of age, they can give consent for their child, if they are capable to give that consent. [21] Refers to national medical research act, where the minor is under 16 years, but in other cases, the minor is under 18 years. Assent – Children since 7 years of age are capable to give their own assent. Assent – Children between 12 and 14 years may have similar competence to give consent as adults. Consent – 16-years.

---

[65] Modi, N., Vohra, J., Preston, J., Elliott, C., Van't Hoff, W., Coad, J., Gibson, F., Partridge, L., Brierley, J., Larcher, V., Greenough, A., Working Party of the Royal College of Paediatrics and Child Health (2014): *Guidance on clinical research involving infants, children and young people: an update for researchers and research ethics committees*, in: Archives of Disease in Childhood 99 (10), 887–891.

[66] McIntosh, N., Bates, P., Brykczynska, G., Dunstan, G., Goldman, A., Harvey, D., Larcher, V., McCrae, D., McKinnon, A., Patton, M., Saunders, J., Shelly, P. (2000): *Guidelines for the ethical conduct of medical research involving children. Royal College of Paediatrics, Child Health: Ethics Advisory Committee*, in: Archives of Disease in Childhood 82 (2), 177–182.

[67] Medical Research Council (2004): *(MRC) Ethics Guide. Medical research involving children*, UK Medical Research Council, London (UK). URL http://www.mrc.ac.uk/documents/pdf/medical-research-involving-children/ [29 August 2017].

EU Commission ad hoc group – Ethical Considerations for Clinical Trials on Medicinal Products Conducted with the Paediatric Population (2008)[68] Revision 1 Published 18Sep2017[69]	"A child", "A minor" and "Pediatric population" mentioned with legal references and ICH E11; Pediatric population between birth and 18 yrs, a child or minor from birth until the legal age of adulthood (usually 18 yrs, rarely 16 yrs.)	Children under 3 yrs; not possible to obtain assent. From 3 yrs ->some capacity of understanding, from 10 yrs >may able to understand information. Assent in writing when a child is able to read and write (about 6-7 yrs ->).	Assent – Children below 3 years; not possible to give own assent. Children since 10 years of age understand given information. Assent – in written form when child is capable to read and write (approx. 6-7 years).
EU – Pediatric Regulation (2007)[70]	"Paediatric population means that part of the population aged between birth and 18 years".	Not defined.	

---

[68] European Union Commission ad hoc group (2008): *Ethical Considerations for Clinical Trials on Medicinal Products Conducted with the Paediatric Population. Recommendations of the Ad hoc group for the development of implementing guidelines for Directive 2001/20/EC relating to good clinical practice in the conduct of clinical trials on medicinal products for human use*. 06 October 2008.URL https://ec.europa.eu/health//sites/health/files/files/eudralex/vol-10/ethical_considerations_en.pdf [29 August 2017].

[69] European Commission (2017): *Ethical considerations for clinical trials on medicinal products conducted with the minors. Recommendations of the expert group on clinical trials for the implementation of Regulation (EU) No 536/2014 on clinical trials on medicinal products for human use. Revision 1 18 September 2017*, in: EudraLex – Volume 10 Clinical trials guidelines, Chapter V, Additional Information. URL https://ec.europa.eu/health/sites/health/files/files/eudralex/vol-10/2017_09_18_ethical_consid_ct_with_minors.pdf [30 October 2017].

[70] European Union (2006): *Regulation (EC) No 1901/2006 of the European Parliament and of the Council of 12 December 2006 on medicinal products for paediatric use and amending Regulation (EEC) No 1768/92, Directive 2001/20/EC, Directive 2001/83/EC and Regulation (EC) No 726/2004*, in: Official Journal of the European Union, L 378/1, 27 December 2006. URL http://ec.europa.eu/health/files/eudralex/vol-1/reg_2006_1901/reg_2006_1901_en.pdf [29 August 2017].

EU – Clinical Trials Regulation (2014)[71] (Expected to be fully implemented during the year 2019).	"A minor" (32), Article 2, 2. (18) according to the law of Member State, and Article 32, 1., "Vulnerable population / minors" Article 10, 1. and "A subject not able to give informed consent" Article 29, 1., 2. "Incapasitated subject" Article 2, 2. (19). Legal age refers to national legislation.	Article 29, 7.,8.: "This Regulation is without prejudice to national law requiring that both the signature of the incapacitated person and the signature of his or her legally designated representative may be required on the informed consent form." and "This Regulation is without prejudice to national law requiring that, in addition to the informed consent given by the legally designated representative, a minor who is capable of forming an opinion and assessing the information given to him or her, shall also assent in order to participate in a clinical trial." Article 32, 1 (b), 2. and 3.; "The minor shall take part in the informed consent procedure in a way adapted to his or her age and mental maturity." AND "If during a clinical trial the minor reaches the age of legal competence to give informed consent as defined in the law of the Member State concerned, his or her express informed consent shall be obtained before that subject can continue to participate in the clinical trial."	

---

[71] European Union (2014): *Regulation EU No 536/2014 of the European Parliament and of the Council of 16 April 2014 on clinical trials on medicinal products for human use*, and repealing *Directive 2001/20/EC. 16 June 2014* (will become applicable no earlier than 28 May 2016). URL http://ec.europa.eu/health/human-use/clinical-trials/regulation/index_en.htm [29 August 2017].

EU Commission – Detailed guidance on the application format and documentation for Ethics Committees opinion (2006)[72]	Age definitions of "a minor" refers to national legislation.	Paragraph 4.6. (page 6–7). says: In trials with minors or incapacitated subjects the procedures to obtain assent/consent from the minor or incapacitated subject, where appropriate, as well as from the parent(s) or legal representative should be described. The notion of legal representative refers back to national legislation. In those cases, two sets of information sheets might be needed according to national regulations. In addition to the information given to the subject's parent(s) or legal representative, the subject should be given information according to his/her capacity to understand. This information should include, where appropriate, a statement that the subject's decision not to participate or to withdraw from a trial will be respected, even if consent is given by the parent/legal representative.	

---

[72] European Commission (2006): *Detailed guidance on the application format and documentation for Ethics Committees opinion on the clinical trial on medicinal products for human use*, in: EudraLex – Volume 10 Clinical trials guidelines, Chapter I: Application and Application Form. URL http://ec.europa.eu/health/documents/eudralex/vol-10/index_en.htm [29 August 2017].

Protection of Minors in Research under the new European Union Regulations

Scarlett JANSEN

A. Introduction

In the recent past the European Union has addressed the topic of human subject research several times. Following the replacement of Directive 2001/20/EC[1] by the regulation on medicinal products for human use[2], a regulation on medical devices[3] has now also been adopted. Both regulations are now in force.[4] The regulation on medicinal products for human use is not expected to be applicable before 2019, as its applicability is linked to the establishment of an EU portal.[5] According to Article 123 (2), the regulation on medical devices will apply from May 26, 2020.[6] Both regulations also contain provisions for research on minors. Because minors are usually not capable to provide consent, this creates the problem of having to legitimize research by means other than personal informed consent. This is similar to situations involving disabled persons, emergency patients and patients unable to provide consent due to illness. This article examines the necessary requirements for legitimate research on minors. After providing an overview of the requirements set out in the regulations (B.), two criteria will be explored in more detail.

---

[1] Directive 2001/20/EC of the European Parliament and of the Council of 4 April 2001 on the approximation of the laws, regulations and administrative provisions of the Member States relating to the implementation of good clinical practice in the conduct of clinical trials on medicinal products for human use (OJ EU L 121/34).

[2] Regulation (EU) No 536/2014 of the European Parliament and of the Council of 16 April 2014 on clinical trials on medicinal products for human use, and repealing Directive 2001/20/EC, (OJ EU L 158/1 of May 27, 2014).

[3] Regulation (EU) 2017/745 of the European Parliament and of the Council of 5 April 2017 on medical devices, amending Directive 2001/83/EC, Regulation (EC) No 178/2002 and Regulation (EC) No 1223/2009 and repealing Council Directives 90/385/EEC and 93/42/EEC (OJ EU L 117/1 of May 5, 2017).

[4] Article 99 of the regulation on medicinal products for human use and Article 123 (1) of the regulation on medical devices.

[5] According to SFL Services, commissioned by the Swiss Federal Office of Public Health to report on the status of implementation of EU Regulation No 536/2014 on clinical trials on medicinal products for human use (updated August 2017, URL https://www.bag.admin.ch/bag/en/home/themen/mensch-gesundheit/biomedizin-forschung/forschung-am-menschen/klinische-pruefungen-humanarzneimitteln-eu.html [27 September 2017].

[6] Article 123 (2) of the regulation on medical devices.

First, in what extent the consent by a legal representative can replace personal consent (C.). Second, which benefit to the individual is required (D.). Finally, a conclusion (E.) will be drawn.

B. Research on Minors under the Regulations

I. The Regulation on Medicinal Products for Human Use

Building on the general requirements of Articles 28 and 29 on the protection of patients and subjects[7], the regulation sets out special requirements for vulnerable persons. The regulation distinguishes between minors and other individuals unable to give consent. While both are unable to provide consent, the former is unable to do so due to his or her age.[8] In making this distinction, the regulation indirectly assumes that the member states set limits on the age from which a person is able to provide consent.[9] However, the definitions fail to recognize that a person's ability to provide consent not only depends on their age, but must also be determined on the basis of their individual circumstances, especially with regard to the complexity of the intervention, its risks and consequences, and the alternatives available. Accordingly, as the risks and possible consequences of medical intervention increase, so do the requirements for ability to provide consent.[10] A rigid age limit, regardless of the type of intervention, would therefore conflict with the right to self-determination.[11]

The requirements for minors are set out in Article 32 of the regulation. Informed consent must have been obtained from the minor's legally designated representative (designated under national law)[12], and the minor must be informed in an appropriate way and involved in the information process.[13] His or her veto

---

[7] For further details, see: Jansen, S. (2016a): *Der Schutz der Patienten und Probanden bei klinischen Prüfungen nach den geplanten Neuerungen im Arzneimittelrecht*, in: Medizinrecht 2016, 417–423, 418f.

[8] See Article 2 Nos. 18, 19 of the regulation on medicinal products for human use.

[9] Jansen 2016a, 417, 419; Jansen, S. (2016b): *Fremdnützige Forschung – ein Tabubruch bei einwilligungsunfähigen Personen? Eine Analyse anlässlich der neuen Verordnung 536/2014 und des Gesetzesentwurfs der Bundesregierung*, in: Lanzerath, D. (ed.): Forschungsethik und klinische Forschung, 57–74, 62.

[10] Amelung, K. (1992): *Über die Einwilligungsfähigkeit (Teil II)*, in: Zeitschrift für die gesamte Strafrechtswissenschaft, 821–833, 833; Geilen, G. (1963): *Einwilligung und ärztliche Aufklärungspflicht*, Bielefeld, 90; Neyen, W. (1991): *Die Einwilligungsfähigkeit im Strafrecht*, Trier, 45.

[11] Jansen, S. (2015): *Forschung an Einwilligungsunfähigen*, Berlin, 42; Wölk, F. (2001): *Der minderjährige Patient in der ärztlichen Behandlung*, in: Medizinrecht 2001, 80–89, 81.

[12] Recital 27 of the regulation on medicinal products for human use; Recital 72 of the regulation on medical devices.

[13] Article 32 (1) lit. a), b), (2) of the regulation on medicinal products for human use.

must be respected.[14] Additionally, no financial or other kind of incentive apart from compensation may be provided.[15] Further, requirements are set out for the clinical trial: Its goal must be to investigate treatments for a medical condition that only occurs in minors or the clinical trial must be essential with respect to minors to validate data obtained in clinical trials on persons able to give informed consent or by other research methods.[16] The clinical trial must also either relate directly to a medical condition from which the minor concerned suffers or be of such a nature that it can only be carried out on minors.[17] In this way, it satisfies the requirement of subsidiarity in that research is only to be carried out on minors if it cannot be carried out with other individuals able to provide consent. It is worth noting in particular the regulation regarding benefit: There must be an expectation that participation in the clinical trial will result in either a *direct benefit* for the minor concerned outweighing the risks and burdens involved, or a benefit for the population represented by the minor concerned and that such a clinical trial will pose only minimal risk to, and will impose minimal burden on, the minor concerned in comparison with the standard treatment of the minor's condition.[18] As such, the regulation considers not only individual benefit, but also *group benefit* to be sufficient. On this basis, it is sufficient that, even if the research does not benefit the person himself or herself, it benefits a group of individuals to which that person belongs to.[19] This notion of group benefit is especially important if no individual benefit is expected, because the patient concerned has already recovered, grown out of the age group in question[20] or died when the research results are released. Group benefit can be considered as a form of third-party benefit,[21] as the group members are unknown to the subject.

---

[14] Article 32 (1) lit. c) of the regulation on medicinal products for human use.
[15] Article 32 (1) lit. d) of the regulation on medicinal products for human use.
[16] Article 32 (1) lit. e) of the regulation on medicinal products for human use.
[17] Article 32 (1) lit. f) of the regulation on medicinal products for human use.
[18] Article 32 (1) lit. g) of the regulation on medicinal products for human use.
[19] See Section 41 (1) No. 2, (2) No. 2 lit. a German Medicinal Products Act (Arzneimittelgesetz – AMG), in: German Federal Law Gazette I, December 12, 2005, 3394; Article 17 of the 'Bioethics Convention', Convention for the Protection of Human Rights and Dignity of the Human Being with regard to the Application of Biology and Medicine: Convention on Human Rights and Biomedicine, URL https://www.coe.int/en/web/conventions/full-list/-/conventions/rms/090000168007cf98 [23 August 2016]; not signed by Germany, for ratification status, see URL https://www.coe.int/en/web/conventions/full-list/-/conventions/treaty/164/signatures [11 October 2017].
[20] See Irmer, F. (2010): *Klinische Forschung mit Nichteinwilligungsfähigen*, Marburg, 15; Jansen 2015, 31.
[21] Graf von Kielmansegg, S. (2008): *Das Prinzip des Eigennutzens in der klinischen Arzneimittelprüfung*, in: Pharma-Recht 2008, 517–525, 518; Jansen 2016b, 57, 60.

Unlike in the case of adults unable to provide consent, in the case of minors, there is no exemption clause with regard to required benefits. Consequently, it is not permissible to impose more stringent national regulations that preclude research with group benefits.[22] While the exemption clause for adults unable to provide consent can be seen as a compromise due to the discussions[23] conducted during the regulation's development phase,[24] group benefit was already included for minors in Directive 2001/20/EC and so no new criticism was made here.

II. The Regulation on Medical Devices

Article 65 of the regulation on medical devices largely parallels the aforementioned requirements of the regulation on medicinal products for human use with regard to research on minors. However, one major difference is that it requires direct benefit for the minor; group benefit is insufficient.[25]

C. Inclusion of Minors in Clinical Trials through Consent

Informed consent is generally accepted as providing legitimacy for medical treatment interfering physical integrity. This also applies to medical research, as derived, for example, from Articles 25ff. of the Declaration of Helsinki. Consequently, for persons unable to provide consent, the question arises if they can be included in clinical trials and how to replace their personal consent in order to include them in research without exploiting them in the process. In this regard, consent by a representative, a veto right and additional approval by the minor are potential options.

---

[22] According to Article 31 (2) of the regulation on medicinal products for human use. Germany has taken note of the exemption clause and, in line with Section 40b (4) sentence 3 AMG, which has not yet entered into force, only permits research with group benefits on adult persons unable to provide consent if consent is anticipated.

[23] In the first draft of the regulation, individual benefit should be retained, see COM(2012) 369 final, Article 30 (1) lit. h of the regulation. According to the report by the Committee on Environment, Public Health and Food Safety (ENVI), an exemption should also be made in the event of low risk, as the regulation only applies to clinical trials with risks, see A7-0208/2013, Amendment 173 (Justification).

[24] Jansen 2016b, 57, 63.

[25] Article 65 lit. g) of the regulation on medical devices.

I. Consent by a Legal Representative

The key requirement for the involvement of minors in research is consent by a legal representative. Under German law, this is usually the minor's parents.[26] Legal representation by parents in particular serves alongside education to enable the minor to participate despite his or her restricted capabilities. The goal here is to expand the scope for action by minors and, as far as possible, achieve legal equality with persons capable of providing consent themselves.[27] Consequently, representation of a minor by his or her parents, who usually know him or her best, most closely approximates to his or her personal consent and can replace it.

However, legitimation by representation has its limits, which according to German law are to be viewed particularly in the interests of the child's welfare.[28] These restrictions ensure that the child is never subject to the arbitrariness of a legal representative. Research with group or third-party benefits is frequently rejected due to incompatibility with the child's welfare.[29] In any case, compatibility with the child's welfare cannot be claimed on the basis that the child, through participation in research with group benefits, is being educated to altruistic action,[30] as education can be provided by more moderate means without infringing upon a child's physical integrity.[31] The link to the child's welfare does not make the child medically untouchable.[32] Representation by parents should enable the child to develop in such a way that interventions to which the child would consent if he or she were able are permitted. Representation of the minor also allows non-indicated interventions to be covered by the principle of the minor's welfare.[33] In this respect, value-related interests such as altruism can also be included in the

---

[26] Sections 1626 and 1629 of the German Civil Code (BGB), in: German Federal Law Gazette I, January 2, 2002, 42, 2909.
[27] Compare in this regard to those receiving care: Jansen 2015, 123ff.
[28] In fact, following a decision by the German Federal Constitutional Court, the welfare of the child even has constitutional status: German Federal Constitutional Court (2002), case no. 1 BvR 1069/01, in: Entscheidungen des Bundesverfassungsgerichts, hg. von den Mitgliedern des Bundesverfassungsgerichts, Tübingen, Vol. 24, 119, 144; Vol. 68, 176, 188; Vol. 72, 155, 172.
[29] Simply see Freund, G. (2013): *Sections 40-42b AMG, Recital 38*, in: Joecks, W., Miebach, K.: Münchener Kommentar zum StGB, Vol. 6, 2nd Edition, Munich; Schimikowski, P. (1980): *Experimente am Menschen*, Stuttgart, 21f.
[30] Though this is asserted by Eberbach, W. (1982): *Die zivilrechtliche Beurteilung der Humanforschung*, Frankfurt a. M., 16f.; Eck, B. (2005): *Die Zulässigkeit medizinischer Forschung mit einwilligungsunfähigen Personen und ihre verfassungsrechtlichen Grenzen*, Frankfurt a. M., 160, although it is stated that this should be restricted to interventions that do not cause bodily injury; von Freier, F. (2009): *Recht und Pflicht der medizinischen Humanforschung*, Heidelberg, p. 85ff.
[31] See Jansen 2015, 134.
[32] Jansen 2015, 139.
[33] Ibid.

process of determining the child's welfare, as long as the related risks and burdens remain very small.[34] Consequently, if their child's stage of development permits, parents have to assess[35] their child's attitude to research measures benefiting third parties and, if possible, decide accordingly as their child's representatives. The more advanced the minor's development, the more likely the child has a point of view and the more readily he or she can be asked about these opinions. To this end, the informed consent discussion provides a framework in which the minor must be involved in any case as far as possible, especially through information. In this way, it is possible to respect the minor's right to self-determination, even in the event of research benefiting third parties, by means of a legal representative and at the same time protect the minor from utilization.

II. Veto

Both regulations mention the minor's right of veto. Article 29 of the Declaration of Helsinki also assumes that heed will be given to a negative decision on the part of the minor. The English version of both regulations states that the minor's right of veto is "respected". However, while the German version of the regulation on medicinal products for human use states that the minor's veto must be merely respected ("respektiert"), it states that the same right for adults unable to provide consent must be heeded ("beachtet"). And the regulation on medical devices states that, for both adults and minors unable to provide consent, this right must be heeded ("beachtet"). Terminology should have been consistent here. The right of veto must be equally relevant for both groups of those unable to provide consent. This is necessitated not only by the right to self-determination, but also by the principal of equality before the law, because minors and adults unable to provide consent have to be treated in the same way in this respect.[36] The use of inconsistent terminology in this context leads to legal uncertainty.[37]

Especially in case of research with group and third-party benefits, a duty to tolerate would violate the dignity of the person unable to provide consent, unless this person had a right of veto.[38] Only in case of medical interventions with an individual benefit for the person concerned and in which there is danger to life

---

[34] Ibid, 142ff.
[35] Ibid, 160.
[36] Jansen 2016b, 57, 69; Jansen 2015, 334 and 239f. (on the Charter of Fundamental Rights:); contrast with Art. 4 lit. c Directive 2001/20/EC, which speaks in of "considered" of the veto right, and the draft regulations, see COM(2012) 369 final, Article 31 (1) lit. c, where account is to be taken based on the subject's age and level of maturity; A7-0208/2013, Amendment 178, Article 31 (1) lit. c.
[37] Jansen 2016, 417, 420.
[38] Jansen 2015, 155.

would it be right to recognize compulsory treatment as an emergency limit under strict conditions.[39] Justice is done to this particular significance of the right of veto if it is made clear that observing it is a fundamental requirement. The requirements for the ability to formulate a negative response in this context are lesser than those for the ability to provide consent,[40] because it is the action which needs to be legitimated, not the stop of the treatment.[41] It is considered sufficient if the person exercising their right to veto is serious in their volition and does not revoke this right.[42] Whether or not the negative decision is plausible or justifiable should be irrelevant.[43]

III. Assent

In addition to the consent of a legal representative, the minor's assent comes into question. Even if he or she is not able to provide consent, it is possible to demand an additional approval by the minor, an assent. This is assumed, for example, under Article 29 of the Declaration of Helsinki. This strengthens the right to self-determination. Neither of the regulations contains provisions on assent. The need for assent gives rise to uncertainty concerning the question which requirements would need to be placed on the ability to provide assent.[44] At the same time, minors unable to provide consent are unable to understand the intervention, assess its implications and make a decision on this basis.[45] Consequently, it should be considered sufficient to heed the right of the minor to veto. In this way, sufficient account is taken of his or her right to self-determination.[46]

---

[39] Amelung, K. (1995): *Vetorechte beschränkt Einwilligungsfähiger in Grenzbereichen medizinischer Intervention*, Berlin, 22ff.; see also Böse, M. (2011): *Zur Rechtfertigung von Zwangsbehandlungen einwilligungsunfähiger Erwachsener*, 523–536, in: Heinrich, M., Jäger, C. (eds.): Festschrift für Claus Roxin zum 80. Geburtstag, 528; see. also German Federal Constitutional Court (BVerfG), decision of July 26, 2016, 1 BvL 8/15, NJW 2017, 53, 55; see also § 1906a BGB.

[40] Amelung 1992, 821, 832; Böse 2011, 523, 529f.; Golbs, U. (2006): *Das Vetorecht eines einwilligungsunfähigen Patienten*, Baden-Baden, 198.

[41] Böse, M. (2017): *Zwischen Selbstbestimmung und Fürsorge: Zwangsbehandlung einwilligungsunfähiger Patienten*, 71–96, in: Revue de Droit Compare Vol. LI No. 1 2017, 81.

[42] Jansen 2015, 158.

[43] Though this is asserted by Golbs 2006, 198f.

[44] See Section 2 (2) of the "Marburger Richtlinien zur Forschung mit einwilligungsunfähigem und beschränkt einwilligungsfähigen Personen" (Marburg guidelines on research with persons unable to provide consent or limited in their capacity to do so) by the Kommission für Ethik in der ärztlichen Forschung (commission for ethics in medical research) at Phillips-Universität Marburg, printed in Freund, G., Heubel, F. (1997): *Forschung mir einwilligungsunfähigen und beschränkt einwilligungsfähigen Personen*, in: Medizinrecht 1997, 347–340, 348ff.

[45] Jansen 2015, p. 159.

[46] Ibid.

IV. Co-consent

Another issue for consideration in addition to the right of veto and the principle of assent is the question of co-consent. This involves obtaining consent from the minor capable of providing such consent and from their legal representative.[47] The regulations on medical devices and medicinal products for human use are without prejudice to national law requiring that, in addition to the informed consent given by the legal representative, a minor shall also assent in order to participate in a clinical trial if he or she is capable of forming an opinion and assessing the information given to him or her.[48] German law provides for a co-consent under medicinal product and medical device legislation.[49] However, the requirement for a person capable of providing consent to do so should actually be self-evident, even if that person is still a minor.[50] If the minor himself or herself is capable of providing consent, the need for additional consent from a representative is a paternalistic measure that devalues the minor's right to self-determination.[51] If the minor is developed in a way that he or she is even able to provide consent for medical research measures, then he or she no longer requires the protection of his or her parents, as this would represent pure heteronomy. Consequently, the minor should have access to a right of sole decision if he or she is capable of providing consent.[52] However, because the regulations focus on minority rather than ability to provide consent, this is not a feasible option. As such, it is pleasing to see that there is at least the possibility of the minor providing additional consent where he or she is capable of doing so, provided national legislation permits this.

---

[47] For this requirement: Lipp, V. (2000): *Freiheit und Fürsorge, Der Mensch als Rechtsperson; zu Funktion und Stellung der rechtlichen Betreuung im Privatrecht*, Tübingen, 34; Olzen, D. (2017): *Section 1666 BGB, Recital 79*, in: Säcker, F., Rixecker, R.: Münchener Kommentar zum Bürgerlichen Gesetzbuch, 7th Edition, Munich; by contrast: Jansen 2015, 147ff.; Odenwald, S. (2004): *Die Einwilligungsfähigkeit im Strafrecht unter besonderer Hervorhebung ärztlichen Handelns*, Frankfurt a. M., 155ff.; Schmidt-Elsaeßer, E. (1988): *Medizinische Forschung an Kindern und Geisteskranken – Zur Strafbarkeit von Forschungseingriffen an Einwilligungsunfähigen*, Frankfurt a. M., 219ff.

[48] Article 63 (7) of the regulation on medical devices and Article 29 (8) of the regulation on medicinal products for human use.

[49] Section 40 (4) No. 3 sentence 4 AMG; Section 20 (4) No. 4 sentence 2 German Medical Devices Act (Medizinproduktegesetz – MPG), in: German Federal Law Gazette I, August 7, 2002, 3146.

[50] Jansen 2015, 335.

[51] See Jansen 2015, 147ff.; Seizinger, K. (1976): *Der Konflikt zwischen dem Minderjährigen und seinem gesetzlichen Vertreter bei der Einwilligung in den Heileingriff im Strafrecht*, Tübingen, 83; Schmidt-Elsaeßer 1988, 223.

[52] Belling, D. W., Eberl, C., Michlik, F. (1994): *Das Selbstbestimmungsrecht Minderjähriger bei medizinischen Eingriffen: eine rechtsvergleichende Studie zum amerikanischen, englischen, französischen und deutschen Recht*, Neuwied 126, 135; Jansen 2015, 153; Schmidt-Elsaeßer 1988, 219.

D. The Benefit to the Individual as a Criterion for Admissibility

In addition to the surrogate for personal consent, it is also worth paying particular attention to the required benefit to the minor, as the regulations differ on this point and research on persons unable to provide consent that benefits third parties is viewed with suspicion.[53] While the regulation on medicinal products for human use extends research with group benefits to adult persons unable to provide consent (even though it does so with an exemption clause), thereby expanding options for research, the requirements of medical device legislation for research on persons unable to provide consent remain high, necessitating an individual benefit. One can only speculate on the reasons for such differentiation. Seemingly, the need for research in this area was not considered to be as high as in the medicinal product sector, where there was a desire to counteract off label use in research with group benefits.[54] Under medicinal product legislation, research on minors with group benefits was already permissible under Directive 2001/20/EC. International guidelines also regularly do not restrict research on minors to research with individual benefits. For example, the Bioethics Convention[55] and the Declaration of Helsinki[56] permit research with group benefits, and the ICH GCP Guidelines even allow research with third-party benefits[57]. By representing the minor and observing the aforementioned protection measures, no conflict arises with the dignity of the minor, as his or her interests are upheld.[58]

Nevertheless, the question still arises as to whether group benefit is a suitable criterion for distinguishing permissible research from research which should not be permitted. There is no relevant difference between group benefit and third-party benefit. Even group benefits do not improve the person's position, as he or she does not benefit from the research his or herself.[59] For the individual themselves, it is immaterial which other individuals benefit from the research. Even reference

---

[53] Simply see von Freier 2009, 85ff.; see also the discussion about the Bioethics Convention: Eser, A. (1996): *Darf nur sein, was einem selber nutzt?*, in: Frankfurter Allgemeine Zeitung, Nov. 19, 1996, No. 270, 16; Rössler, D. (1996): *Zur Diskussion über die Bioethik-Konvention*, in: Ethik in der Medizin 1996, 167–172; Spranger, T. M. (2000): *Fremdnützige Forschung an Einwilligungsunfähigen*, in: Sozialrecht und Praxis 2000, 71–79.
[54] On the AMG: Bundestags-Drucksachen 15/2109, 31.
[55] Article 17 (2) of the Bioethics Convention.
[56] Article 28 of the WMA Declaration of Helsinki – Ethical Principles for Medical Research Involving Human Subjects, German version available at http://www.bundesaerztekammer.de/fileadmin/user_upload/Deklaration_von_Helsinki_2013_DE.pdf [11 October 2017].
[57] Article 4.8.13 of the Guideline for Good Clinical Practice E6(R1), available at https://www.ich.org/fileadmin/Public_Web_Site/ICH_Products/Guidelines/Efficacy/E6/E6_R1_Guideline.pdf [11 October 2017].
[58] Jansen 2015, 114ff.
[59] Jansen 2016a, 417, 420; ibid. 2016b, 57, 61.

to a particular feeling of solidarity[60] does not justify differentiation. Any special feeling of solidarity would have to be demonstrated in the individual case.[61] The same applies to the assumption that the person would be likely to provide consent if he or she could, given that he or she shares the same fate as those the research would benefit.[62] The sense of solidarity could also apply to other persons as well as to those who belong to the group in question, for example, ill family members.[63] The characteristic of group benefit is arbitrary, as illustrated by the wide range of options for group formation.[64] One can justify membership of a group by age, illness or capability, or even by inability to provide consent.[65] Finally, group membership could be applied to all people who could be helped through the research.[66] The criterion of group benefit should serve to prevent patients unable to provide consent from being exploited for research purposes.[67] Research should only be conducted with such persons if there is no other alternative available. This is precisely what the characteristic of subsidiarity achieves. Provided the subsidiarity of research on those unable to provide consent as opposed to research on those able to provide consent is taken seriously, there is no need for the restrictive and rather arbitrary characteristic of group benefit.[68] The regulations particularly stress the fact that the goal of clinical trials must be to research treatments for medical conditions that only affect minors or that these trials must be essential to confirm data relating to minors. This serves to counteract the utilization of minors. In conjunction with the other protection mechanisms provided for by the regulations, minors are protected, yet can still be involved in research.

E. Conclusion

The regulations largely satisfy the requirements for research involving minors. They assume the provision of consent by a legal representative. Such representative consent can also provide legitimacy for research with group benefits that is permissible in the context of research into medicinal products. The right to veto should fundamentally be observed on a binding basis. The need to heed this veto

---

[60] Helmchen, H., Lauter, H. (eds.) (1995): *Ärzte mit Demenzkranken forschen? – Analyse des Problemfeldes Forschungsbedarf und Einwilligungsproblematik*, Stuttgart, New York, 28.
[61] Jansen 2016a, 417, 420; ibid. 2016b, 57, 62.
[62] Rosenau, H. (2006): *Bioethik (J)*, in: Heun, W., Honecker, M., Morlok, M., Wieland, J. (eds.): Evangelisches Staatslexikon, column 222.
[63] Jansen 2015, 166; ibid. 2016a, 417, 420.
[64] Jansen 2015, 167f.; ibid. 2016a, 417, 420; ibid. 2016b, 57, 62.
[65] Irmer, F. 2010, 9; Magnus, D. (2006): *Medizinische Forschung an Kindern*, Tübingen, 63.
[66] Jansen 2016a, 417, 420.
[67] Jansen 2015, S. 167f.; ibid., 2016a, 417, 420.
[68] Jansen 2015, 168.; ibid. 2016a, 417, 420; ibid. 2016b, 57, 62.

could be expressed more clearly in the different language versions. Assent is not necessary. The regulations do not assume the possibility of minors capable of providing consent being able to provide sole consent to participating in the research measures. Nevertheless, there is the possibility of minors providing additional consent where national regulations permit. Minors are also protected by additional protection measures. Subsidiarity is extremely important in this context, as it can prevent utilization. The criterion of group benefit by contrast appears arbitrary.

Ethical Issues on Research with Minors and Challenges for Research Ethics Committees

Dirk LANZERATH

Introduction

Ethically sound research protocols involving children assume that ethics includes much more than procedural compliance with a prescribed set of rules or codes of conduct that should guarantee good or safe research in any given context. The requirements of ethical research with minors extend beyond a formal involvement of a research ethics committee (REC) or an institutional review board (IRB).[1] Rather, ethics in research is related to the attitudes, beliefs, and habits of the researchers involved that are based on reliable social norms, and which constitute trusted research within a complex social environment. Compared to research with adults – as always when we interact with children in and outside of research and diagnostic and therapeutic praxis – we need to consider the whole system where a child or an adolescent is involved: the *family*, the *institutions*, the *society*. Here is the node where RECs have an important role, one that is often considered as an *intermediary role* between science and society and between the legal and political systems.[2] This role is more or less specified by professional law or soft law. However, this specific role needs to be reflected against the background of various cultural and social concerns confronted with a variety of interests and influences – implicitly and explicitly: There are the children themselves, the parents or guardians, the sponsor, the peer group, the community, the tribe, the more collectively or more individualistically organized societies, and many other groups and stakeholders involved.[3]

The interpretation how to *reflect* and how to *respect* fundamental ethical principles such as autonomy, beneficence, non-maleficence, justice, or solidarity might differ along with their priorities and hierarchies. None of them can be easily transferred from the debate on research with adults to research with children

---

[1] In this paper I use only the expression research ethics committee (REC), even if there are national or regional differences.
[2] Schomberg, R. von (2007): *From the Ethics of Technology towards an Ethics of Knowledge Policy & Knowledge Assessment. A working document from the European Commission Services*, Brussels.
[3] Cf. Graham, A., Powell, M., Taylor, N., Anderson, D., Fitzgerald, R. (2013): *Ethical Research Involving Children (ERIC)*, UNICEF Office of Research – Innocenti, Florence, 2, 13.

because children do not have the same level of autonomy, awareness, or experience and they belong to a very vulnerable group that needs and expects various levels of *protection* and *participation*. Moreover, the group of children is not a homogeneous group and needs differentiated attention according to their individual degree of maturity. Therefore "ethical considerations have shifted significantly from a predominant focus on protectionist discourses, which positioned children as vulnerable and requiring safeguarding by adults including researchers, to an emphasis on recognising children's agency and competency, and highlighting children's participation rights. Both dimensions are critically important to children's well-being, however these can, at times, present as contradictory and/or opposing. [. . .] Rather than being seen in oppositional terms, children's protection and participation are viewed such that the competence, dependence and vulnerability of children do not, in themselves, determine their inclusion or exclusion from research so much as inform the way in which their participation takes place. [. . .] Hence, attention is drawn to the important role of dialogue, collaboration and critically reflective practice in navigating the uncertainty that often arises in ethical decision-making."[4] What has to be considered is the practical application of the required ethical principles with regard to harms and benefits, informed consent, privacy, confidentiality, and integration in the decision-making procedure.

1. Respecting Autonomy, Desires, and Capabilities

Respecting autonomy and individual desires is closely linked with rights and duties, and implies valuing children including the context of their lives, and recognizing their dignity. Against this background, the *UNICEF Office of Research* launched the project "Best Practice Requirements by the Ethical Research Involving Children." The project emphasizes that respecting the autonomy of children requires more of an individualized perspective compared to similar research with adults.

Researchers who integrate minors in their studies need to consider the individuality of the child, the cultural context of the child, and how this culture shapes their experiences, desires, capabilities, and perspectives. This is not only relevant for clinical trials or experiments in the biomedical context but also for psychological or sociological studies within the humanities such as interviews and qualitative studies. This perspective considers the various subjective and relational experiences of minors. They are influenced by culture, community, legal backgrounds, peer groups, and others. Ethically sound research takes these perspectives of the social environment, which vary strongly from culture to culture, into account. Re-

---

[4] Graham et al. 2013, 14.

searchers and RECs that consult researchers respect the *unequal relationships of power* between researchers and children, between children and their social environment. These unequal relationships call for a specific communication process between the actors.[5] In particular education, peer groups, and other actors of the social environment have an important impact on the expectations and feelings of the minors who serve as research participants.

2. Beneficence and Non-maleficence

Ethical aspects of beneficence and non-maleficence need not only be considered concerning what researchers *do* when children and adolescents are participants in medical research; it is also important to consider what they *do not do*. When we consider the rights of children, including the obligation that research on children is conducted seriously so that they can benefit from any improvement in health conditions or quality of life, omissions also have to be ethically justified. Opportunities to make progress for the *benefit* of children through research should be taken. A risk–benefit assessment needs to take these options into account against the background of the ethical principle of *beneficence*.

Doing no harm, the principle of non-maleficence, therefore, includes a careful assessment of both acts and non-acts, commissions and omissions. Omissions might also harm children in the long run. Research that includes children has the potential to improve their quality of life, their health, and practices in medical care in general.[6] Inclusion and exclusion both have to be justified. These ethical considerations must not only cover the acts *during* the process of research but also *before* and *after*. *Recruitment* and *data collection and storage* could harm, with an enormous potential for *discrimination and stigmatization* in a much later stage of life – children, adolescents, and their families can often not assess the long-term consequences. The storage of health data may lead to disadvantages later in life, for example in relation to insurance policies or situations at workplaces. Therefore, protecting minors as research participants includes ethical reflections already in the preparatory process before the research starts and needs to be continued in the dissemination phase, in particular when data linked to personal details are stored in a biobank. It is essential to reflect that an ethical assessment is not only

---

[5] Cf. Graham et al. 2013, 15.
[6] Greene, S., Hill, M. (2005): *Researching children's experience: methods and methodological issues*, in: Hogan, D., Greene, S. (eds.): Researching children's experience: Methods and approaches, London, 1–21; Hinton, R., Tisdall, E. K. M., Gallagher, M., Elsley, S. (2008): *Children and young people's participation in public decision-making*, in: International Journal of Children's Rights 16, 281–284.

required for the physical act of research. Conversations, questions, and interviews can cause harm, as can careless handling of confidential knowledge or data.

The principles of beneficence and non-maleficence result in permission or rejection, but it always has to be considered what might happen if the research is not performed. In some cases we might miss out on important scientific and societal opportunities. In patient groups, the advantages of the research usually outweigh the disadvantages. This perception is often a point of conflict between patient groups and the tasks of research ethics committees, whose goal is to protect the research participants. The perception of risks and burdens varies. Parents, children, and members of RECs have different perspectives here. There is a very difficult balance between the benefit of potential therapeutic improvements, protection against significant risks, and overprotection.[7] However, a problem of the relationship between research and medical benefit is that even if researchers avoid causing any harm, they do not know whether their findings will lead to any beneficial results. The results of research cannot be prejudged. This is the nature of science and research.

3. Justice and Solidarity

The principle of justice is one of the fundamental ethical principles in social ethics, medical ethics, and research ethics. In some ethical theories it is considered the central principle and is identified with morality in the sense of "what we owe to each other"[8]. Against this background it often leads to the aspect of "just" procedures. But justice can mean much more when considered as an essential virtue[9] and the natural "sense of justice" can be regarded as a description and indicator of human morality at all.[10] To emphasize the social importance of justice, which is not just reduced to procedural claims, justice is often related to the principle of *solidarity* in European bioethical discussions.[11]

Justice includes many different dimensions and raises various normative questions when it comes to research involving children.[12] The question of *just* and *fair*

---

[7] O'Lonergan, T. A., Milgrom, H. (2005): *Ethical Considerations in Research Involving Children*, in: Current Allergy and Asthma Reports 5, 451–458, 455.
[8] Scanlon, T. (1998): *What We Owe to Each Other*, Cambridge, Mass.
[9] Aristotle (ca. 350): *Ethica Nicomachea*, 1102a-1103a, Ross, W. D. (trans.) (1925): Aristotle. The Nicomachean Ethics. Translated with an Introduction, Oxford.
[10] Cf. Rawls, J. (1999): *A Theory of Justice*, Cambridge, 125.
[11] Cf. ter Meulen, R. (2016): Solidarity, justice, and recognition of the other, in: Theoretical Medicine and Bioethics 37 (6), 517–529, URL https://link.springer.com/content/pdf/10.1007%2Fs11017-016-9387-3.pdf [22 March 2018].
[12] Greig, A. D., Taylor, J., MacKay, T. (2013): *Doing Research with Children. A Practical Guide*, Los Angeles, 16, 253.

acts arises in the relationship between researcher and child and in any dialogue and conversation that takes place between them. The relationship between the child as a research participant and the adult researchers is subject to a *dramatic power difference* between these actors. Therefore the researcher needs to listen respectfully to the views, perspectives, fears, and intentions of the children involved.[13] Giving due weight to these considerations and including children's responses in the design and undertaking of research allows a research process and its results to be considered as just. It reflects the message of the Belmont Report on justice, namely finding the "right balance between the perceived benefits of the research and perceived burdens placed on the participants."[14] The criteria on which participants will be included or excluded in a research protocol are also related to the concept of justice to avoid any kind of discrimination. The selection needs to be related to the research purposes.[15] Reliable research with children takes this into account because science and research are not a separate world but a part of a just social environment with specific relationships between children and adults. Against this background we can identify for this research context a *bilateral sphere of justice* and a *social sphere of justice*. The concept of justice "concerns the (re)distribution of burdens and benefits of research, including consideration of the *allocation of material and social resources* to support the respectful and ethical involvement of children."[16]

This leads to the important aspect of solidarity, which plays a crucial role in ethical considerations justifying this type of research. The International Ethical Guidelines for Health-related Research Involving Humans Prepared by the Council for International Organizations of Medical Sciences (CIOMS) states that the *scientific* and *social value* of health-related research involving humans attains its ethical justification from its scientific and social value. This is considered as the potential of generating the knowledge and the means necessary to protect and promote people's health. "Patients, health professionals, researchers, policy-makers, public health officials, pharmaceutical companies and others rely on the results of research for activities and decisions that impact individual and public health, welfare, and the use of limited resources. Therefore, researchers, sponsors, research ethics committees, and health authorities, must ensure that proposed studies are scientifically sound, build on an adequate prior knowledge base, and are likely to

---

[13] Cf. Graham et al. 2013, 17.
[14] National Commission for the Protection of Human Subjects of Biomedical and Behavioural Research (1979): *The Belmont Report. Ethical principles and guidelines for the protection of human subjects of research.* URL http://ohsr.od.nih.gov/ [15 March 2018].
[15] Cf. Graham et al. 2013, 17.
[16] Fraser, N. (2008):*From redistribution to recognition? Dilemmas of justice in a "postsocialist" age*, in: Olson, K. (ed.): Adding insult to injury: Nancy Fraser debates her Critics, London, 9–41.

generate valuable information. Although scientific and social value are the fundamental justification for undertaking research, researchers, sponsors, research ethics committees and health authorities have a moral obligation to ensure that all research is carried out in ways that uphold human rights, and respect, protect, and are fair to study participants and the communities in which the research is conducted. Scientific and social value cannot legitimate subjecting study participants or host communities to mistreatment, or injustice."[17]

Nevertheless, research is usually not for the benefit or at least not for the direct benefit of the research participant. In the ethically controversial field of research with children, the *benefit of the group* – like the group of those who suffer from the same disease – is an important aspect of social justification. It means it is not completely for the benefit of a strange third party, but also not a direct benefit for the involved subject. This *solidarity* among the fellow sufferers is an important aspect in order to apply the principle of justice. A well-considered concept of justice that takes the mentioned dramatic differences into account includes that children are perceived not as objects but as subjects who can also play a crucial role as *advisors and consultants*. Researchers, RECs, and their members can learn from them to improve their work and performance when working with minors.[18]

4. Informed Consent and Assent

A justified decision-making process involves the process of informed consent and/or assent of the involved human subject. Consent includes an explicit act. It starts with a decision concerning *who* is involved in the act of consent. This depends on the age of the minor, the family situation, and the legal framework (in particular concerning legal custody). The underlying relationships are complex and can usually be described as a triad, in contrast to the common participant/researcher dyad. This triad consists of the *researcher*, *child/adolescent participant*, and *parent* or *guardian*. When the direct consent of a minor is documented it shows the respect for the rights and needs of minors and gives less space for any manipulation by third parties. The consent of the parents or guardians or proxy consent is also an ethical and legal requirement when minors participate in a research protocol. This is the other safety measure to prevent certain manipulations on the researcher's side. How the consent is given depends a lot on the age

---

[17] Council for International Organizations of Medical Sciences (CIOMS) (2016): *International Ethical Guidelines for Health-related Research Involving Humans. Prepared by the Council for International Organizations of Medical Sciences (CIOMS) in collaboration with the World Health Organization (WHO)*, Geneva, 1.

[18] Cf. the chapters of Begonya Nafria Escalera et al., of Jennifer Preston et al., and of Kate Harvey in this volume.

and maturity level.[19] Whatever the parents and guardians decide, the voice of the child has to be respected. The situation is fundamentally different to therapeutic acts where a direct benefit for the minor can be expected.

The concept of informed consent requires a basic understanding of the research concerned. This means that the consent is considered not only as a formal but also as a well-informed agreement. Therefore, a requirement of ethically justified research with human participants is that researchers provide the participants with well-prepared information on the research activity, whatever research methodology is being used. Equally, *children and adolescents must be provided with information that is appropriate to their age and competencies*, bearing in mind the environmental context, differing experiences, and evolving capacities of each minor. Against this backdrop, it becomes clear that the involved children should broadly understand the main objectives of the research and the potential risks, benefits, and burdens. Adequate provided information leads to a meaningful choice and a reliable process before the research starts. This also includes an understanding that there is probably no direct benefit for them.

Adequate information sheets about the research and its objectives, risks, and burdens also have to be prepared for parents or guardians. Researchers should be prepared to talk with them about the role of the minor as a research participant but also about their own position and obligations. "Information can be provided which underlines children's capacity to be involved in research and helps parents to *assist* children to make decisions about taking part, *rather than substituting their own views* or acting on their own convenience, except in situations when the child is unable to express a view or is especially vulnerable. However, to respect children's autonomy, the use of proxy informants should be minimised. The child needs to give informed consent [or assent] as well as the person who is acting as the proxy wherever possible."[20] Assent means that children can legally not give consent but that they voluntarily agree to take part in a study. They may also dissent, which means they do not agree, and this opinion has to be taken seriously even though the consent of the parents or the guardian is necessary. The discussion about assent and consent is not only a legal debate. Apart from the necessity to get the approval of the parents or the guardian, the inclusion of the child's consideration is of ethical importance anyway, if we are to take their autonomy and interests seriously. It is important that children will not be manipulated, although it is difficult to define when *manipulation* starts. Parents know how often children are being manipulated by them when they rebel against necessary medical treatment for their own benefit, but the research situation is completely different. There is

---

[19] Cf. Graham et al. 2013, 57–58.
[20] Cf. Graham et al. 2013, 58.

much more need to respect the child's voice when there is no direct benefit. Due to the dramatic power differences of the actors mentioned above, manipulation may start early with a certain kind of rhetoric. But the aim of the conversation should be truth and trustfulness as part of reliable research.

The way the information materials are presented is of significant importance.

The written signature is the usual way to confirm consent or assent. But in some cultural circumstances thumb prints or even verbal agreements are also accepted. In particular in African countries an individual-based consent model and the use of written consent documents may be problematic. In these places the norms of decision-making do not emphasize individual autonomy and illiteracy rates are high. Therefore several ethical models endorse "the use of community approval and verbal consent for research in countries where cultural values and practices emphasize oral rather than written agreements and where community leaders, elders, and tribal chiefs play an important role in decision-making."[21] Flexible means of providing information and signifying consent are essential for children, or parents, who are not able or willing to use written methods. Signing consent forms can also be problematic and/or intimidating for those who are not physically able to, and for people who are not literate or are particularly vulnerable. When the informed consent should be particularly "informed", the way the information is provided is decisive. The information sheet for minors can be substituted by completely different tools like videos, oral communication, or comic strips. The intention must be that the child has, according to its maturation and capacities, a clear idea about the objectives of the research and the risks and burdens.

5. Privacy and Confidentiality

Already in the planning phase as well as in the data collection phase of a research project the researchers need to respect the privacy and confidentiality of the research participants. This requires a certain kind of awareness and sensibility. The research protocol should contain measures on how information will be kept private and how the data are shared and stored. Long-term anonymization is an important aspect. In the research process itself, the researchers should be flexible and be able to adapt to emerging issues concerning privacy and confidentiality. The communication with the child on how much information they want to share or reveal is of great importance and a sensitive issue. Privacy and the right to be free from intrusion or interference by others is a basic human right also for minors. This includes

---

[21] Onvomaha Tindana, P., Kass, N., Akweongo, P. (2006): *The Informed Consent Process in a Rural African Setting: A Case Study of the Kassena-Nankana District of Northern Ghana*, in: IRB: Ethics & Human Research 28 (3), 1.

a positive relationship with the parents – as long as it is not against the interests of the child. This is a delicate balance that is well known from treatments in medicine and psychotherapy. It is important that a minor knows that the researcher will not disclose information without notifying the child of the need to do so. To decide when parents can be excluded and when not is a difficult assessment.[22]

To take this right of confidentiality seriously, it is important to respect that children share only the information that they wish to when participating in research activities and, if necessary, ensure that they understand that in some circumstances it may be preferable to keep certain information private. The type of data that is collected during research creates various ethical concerns in regard to how much information children wish to share. For example, in biomedical research that involves children, the collection and storage of biological data, such as genetic/DNA information, raises an ethical issue concerning the child's understanding about what will potentially be revealed from providing this type of data. In particular concerning genetic data that is stored, a certain kind of knowledge about individual health risks becomes public or semi-public when the processes of anonymization or pseudonymization are uncertain. A minor cannot foresee the later societal consequences.[23] This is an enormous source of later discrimination and stigmatization. The combination of collecting data from genetics, brain imaging, and psychological interviews on behavior and social context, as has been performed in IMAGEMEND, is a very sensitive procedure. Biological data, health data, and personal data are being combined. The statistical correlations might be an important step for research but open to a variety of interpretations. The data and the correlations could be a source of later discrimination and stigmatization which cannot be foreseen by children and adolescents. Genetic data in particular may also become a challenge for the family system, when a finding about one person also affects relatives of the person concerned. Other persons, including parents, may be interested in the information that has been collected, but the researcher is ethically obliged to treat the information carefully and retain confidentiality related to the maturity level of the minor.

---

[22] Cf. Bruch, H. (2016): *The Role of the Parent in Psychotherapy with Children*, in: Psychiatry, 11 (2), 169–175. URL https://www.tandfonline.com/doi/abs/10.1080/00332747.1948.11022679 [22 March 2018].

[23] Lanzerath, D. (2014): *The Use of Genetic Knowledge*, in: Lanzerath, D., Heinrichs, B., Rietschel, M., Schmäl, C. (eds.): Incidental Findings – Scientific, Legal and Ethical Issues, Bd. 26 (Medizin-Ethik), Köln, 93–108; In gene-based prevention trials, the implications of the disclosure of the test results needs to be fully considered by researchers, disclosed during the consent process and understood by the parents and the children (Spriggs, M. (2010): *Understanding consent in research involving children*, Melbourne).

6. The Challenges for Research Ethics Committees

Against this background it is necessary to identify the challenges for the work of ethics review boards like institutional review boards (IRBs) or research ethics committees (RECs) because their central obligation is to protect the research participants. Considering the globalized world and internationally organized research linked with global players such as big pharma companies, we should expect to find the same ethical standards and ethical review mechanisms everywhere where research is taking place. But even when we can identify some common ethical principles in research ethics such as autonomy, beneficence, non-maleficence, justice, or solidarity, its interpretation and practical implementation vary and differ from region to region and from culture to culture. In the biomedical sector of research there are – at least – some global ethics review mechanisms. Ethics review boards aim to ensure that ethical standards of conduct of research activities are met, and therefore participants are protected from harm. As such, they are a resource that could potentially help researchers in their process of ethical decision-making. The "intermediary role" of RECs as a player between science and society should result in qualified links between the claims of researchers and the demands of a society by protecting the participating individuals.

Apart from international guidelines and regulations like the Declaration of Helsinki, the CIOMS, or ICH guidelines we know that the national regulations, standards, and – in particular – practical procedures quite often vary. At least in Europe RECs should work hard to improve and to adjust their standards and procedures for the ethical review process step by step but by taking into consideration the various cultural differences. The implementation of the Clinical Trial Regulation EU No. 536/2014 might lead to more harmonization procedures among the work of RECs in Europe.

However, we have to realize that the biomedical sector – in particular drug trials – is more advanced concerning consistent ethical reviews than other research areas, especially in empirical humanities. But surveys with interviews and other measures to collect data could also harm research participants – in particular children. This is often underestimated in the scientific community. The critical participation and involvement of IRBs or RECs can critically and productively accompany the research here. The involvement of RECs in the research process has been a great achievement ever since the Nuremberg Trials. Even though the Nuremberg code did not influence the later legislation and proceedings directly, in the time after Nuremberg and later after the Tuskegee Syphilis Study a debate was initiated that resulted in guidelines, legislation, and the establishment of ethics committees to ensure a clear and independent mechanism to protect research participants.

Therefore the ethics committees in Europe were very surprised that after nine years of experience with the European Good Clinical Practice Directive[24] the European Commission presented in 2012 a draft of a new regulation on clinical trials on medicinal products for human use[25] that marginalized the role of ethics committees. It took a lot of lobbying to strengthen this aspect of reviewing biomedical research protocols and to now have an at least acceptable text of the regulation that includes ethics committees not only implicitly.

Looking at various studies, some researchers are critical of the increasingly formal, frustrating regulation. In particular the involvement of RECs is sometimes considered a bureaucratic burden that does not provide a better ethical understanding of the research and that creates formal obstacles and time delays for good research and progress in health and quality of life. In research with minors, RECs are sometimes criticized for their ostensibly overprotective attitude.[26]

Obviously there is a need for more effective exchange between researchers who are involved in research with children and RECs. A critical involvement of RECs should not patronize researchers, but encourage them to develop their own practices to consider aspects in research ethics concerning their own research protocols and projects. Apart from the legal situation and the objective of RECs to protect the research participants, an approval or a favorable opinion of a REC is often mandatory to get research results published in a scientific journal and to receive funds from a funding agency. Scientific journals and funding agencies will be important stakeholders to support a harmonization procedure in establishing review systems outside the realm of drug trials.

The balance between beneficial research and protection of the participants – in particular children and adolescents – is a great challenge for RECs: How are young research participants as a very vulnerable group to be protected while not excluding them from scientific achievements concerning the development of new therapies? This may involve the inclusion of minors in trials where they are legally or physically not able to give consent. The EU regulation clearly opens this path when it states that "a clinical trial on minors may be conducted only where, in addition to the conditions set out in Article 28, all of the following conditions are met: (a) the informed consent of their legally designated representative has been

---

[24] Directive 2005/28/EC of 8 April 2005 of the European Parliament and of the Council.
[25] Regulation (EU) No 536/2014 of the European Parliament and of the Council of 16 April 2014 on clinical trials on medicinal products for human use, and repealing Directive 2001/20/EC.
[26] Cf. Gallagher, M., Haywood, S., Jones, M., Milne, S. (2010): *Negotiating informed consent with children in school-based research: A critical review*, in: Children and Society 24, 471–482; Powell, M., Smith, A. B. (2009): *Children's participation rights in research*, in: Childhood 16, 124–142; Matthys, D., Rose, K. (2010): *Ethics in paediatric research. Three years after introduction of the European Regulation*, in: Rose, K., Van den Anker, J. N. (eds.): Guide to Paediatric Drug Development and Clinical Research, Basel, 71–74.

obtained; (b) the minors have received the information referred to in Article 29(2) in a way adapted to their age and mental maturity […]."[27]

These provisions mean for RECs that they have to assess the scientific grounds for benefits (direct benefit, benefit for the represented group (a specific case of a third-party benefit), examining evidence that it can only be carried out on minors). Ethics committees need to determine whether a provided risk assessment (minimal risk/minimal burden) can be guaranteed by the procedures in the research protocols. With regard to the informed consent procedure RECs have to ensure that the information provided is clearly adapted to the age and mental maturity of the minors. It is also necessary to evaluate the forms of consent, legal representative consent, and assent. The form needs to be much more creative compared to the work with adults. To fulfill these requirements and demands the RECs need to include someone with the experience in that kind of research. That does not mean that researchers shall "pass on ethical responsibility to ethics review committees, who cannot guarantee that ethical research is supported and poor research is prevented."[28]

Generally speaking, the RECs play a significant role in this process but the role is also a very difficult one, because the *players* and *parties* involved are characterized by *very different interests and a variety of distinct backgrounds*:

– *Researchers* involved in research with minors and adolescents have experience with these groups but they also have a scientific interest and interest in a scientific career that might be detached from the interests of the well-being of the research participants.
– *The sponsor* has an interest not to harm people with newly developed drugs but also an interest in financial gains.
– *Parents* concentrate on the well-being of the children but do not have the background to foresee all benefits and risks for the child and often struggle between protection and unrealistic ambition.
– *Patient groups* are a very important group with a lot of experience and background knowledge but they are sometimes influenced by third parties – in particular when they receive direct financial funds from industry.
– *The minors* themselves often don't know how to react and might be overwhelmed by the situation outside their therapeutic conditions; for RECs it is not easy to find proper ways to adapt the informed consent procedure so that it is in accordance with the age and mental maturity of the minors.

---

[27] Regulation (EU) No 536/2014 of the European Parliament and of the Council of 16 April 2014 on clinical trials on medicinal products for human use, and repealing Directive 2001/20/EC.
[28] Alderson, P., Morrow, V. (2011): *The ethics of research with children and young people*, London.

7. Conclusions

RECs reviewing research with children and adolescents should be multidisciplinary and independent. In the context of clinical research with minors, at least one member should have experience in conducting pediatric research.[29] If none of the members have such expertise, the board should seek the advice of an ad hoc expert.[30] The implementation of such recommendations may better position ethics review boards to protect the children and families participating in research and provide valuable, ongoing support for researchers. Whether specific research ethics committees should be established that are focused on considering research with children and young people[31] is a highly controversial question. The inclusion of children, young people, and parent groups in RECs and involving them in the screening of research projects[32] is often recommended, but not often realized. It is important that the children's roles do not have an alibi function and "that the heterogeneity of children is represented."[33] But the effort that has to be made here is very high and well described in this volume.[34] At least the laypeople's perspective on a board should be covered by a representative of the parent group concerned. Additionally it is necessary to offer training opportunities to ensure that REC members have a current understanding of children and their levels of competence.[35] Against this background the Network of Research Ethics Committees (EUREC) has recently been working in close cooperation with the European Network of Paediatric Research at the European Medicines Agency (Enpr-EMA)

---

[29] Cf. Avard, D., Samuel, J., Black, L., Griener, G., Knoppers, B. (2011): *Best practices for health research involving children and adolescents: Genetic, pharmaceutical, longitudinal studies and palliative care research*, The Centre of Genomics and Policy at McGill University, and Ethics Office, Canadian Institutes of Health research; Council for International Organizations of Medical Sciences (CIOMS), World Health Organization (WHO) (2002): *International ethical guidelines for biomedical research involving human subjects*, Geneva; Council for International Organizations of Medical Sciences (CIOMS), World Health Organization (WHO) (2008): *International ethical guidelines for epidemiological studies*, Geneva.

[30] Cf. Avard et al. 2011.

[31] Cf. Powell, Smith 2006; Stalker, K., Carpenter, J., Connors, C., Phillips, R. (2004): *Ethical issues in social research: difficulties encountered gaining access to children in hospital for research*, in: Child: Care, Health and Development 30, 377–383.

[32] Cf. Carter, B. (2009): *Tick box for child? The ethical positioning of children as vulnerable, researchers as barbarians and reviewers as overly cautious*, in: International Journal of Nursing Studies 46, 858–864.; Coyne, I. (2010a): *Research with children and young people: The issue of parental (proxy) consent*, in: Children and Society 24, 227–237.

[33] Carter 2009.

[34] Cf. the chapters of Begonya Nafria Escalera et al., of Jennifer Preston et al., and of Kate Harvey in this volume.

[35] Cf. Campbell, A. (2008): *For their own good: Recruiting children to research*, in: Childhood 15, 30–49; Coyne, I. (2010b): *Accessing children as research participants: Examining the role of gatekeepers*, in: Child: Care, Health and Development 36, 452–454.

in establishing a common working party of researching pediatricians from Enpr-EMA and representatives from RECs. This is to improve the research with minors from a scientific and from an ethical perspective.

RECs play a significant role in the research process and can make a significant contribution not only to preventing bad research but also to protecting research participants. They can also be a buffer between the researchers and the participants. Current research often includes collaborations between researchers from multiple institutions or countries with different regulations. Here, more harmonization is desired. This includes compliance with the requirements of the formal ethics review in countries where the research takes place and compliance with international guidelines. But a serious and growing concern is that research is increasing in countries with lower ethical standards.[36] The Nuffield Council on Bioethics' working party that prepared the report "The ethics of research related to healthcare in developing countries" recommends an effective system of review of the ethical propriety of research because it is a crucial safeguard for participants. The system should include the "establishment and maintenance of research ethics committees that are independent of government and sponsors of research. Research should be subject to ethical review in both the country(ies) hosting and the country(ies) sponsoring the research. The Working Party welcomes international initiatives for establishing research ethics committees, training their members and monitoring their development."[37] Therefore it is also necessary to establish an alliance of ethics committees and ethics committee members beyond EUREC as an international platform of exchange. This could be a basis to develop the right balance between the protection of children as participants in research and progress in research as a benefit for the group.

---

[36] Alderson, Morrow 2011, 74; Alderson, P., Morrow, V. (2004): *Ethics, social research and consulting with children and young people*, London; Balen, R., Blyth, E., Calabretto, H., Fraser, C., Horrocks, C., Manby, M. (2006): *Involving children in health and social research: 'Human becomings' or 'active beings'?*, in: Childhood 13, 29–48.

[37] Nuffield Council on Bioethics (2002): *The ethics of research related to healthcare in developing countries*, xvi.

KIDS Barcelona: Young Persons' Advisory Group Focused in Clinical Research and Innovation Projects

Begonya Nafria Escalera, Joana Claverol Torres

Introduction

Sant Joan de Déu Children's Hospital is the largest paediatric hospital in Spain. We are a healthcare and research organization that includes all therapeutic areas of paediatrics. At the same time, in a close collaboration with all these medical services, we have a clinical trials unit to centralize all the research projects addressed to study innovative treatments.

The principles of our organization are focused to treat the patient and the family under a holistic concept of health. It means that they are at the centre of our activity as active members, helping us to deliver better healthcare services and better research projects. Both areas have a dedicated department to centralize and ensure the participation of patients and families. When we refer to healthcare services the Patient Experience Department is responsible and when we refer to the involvement of patients in research (including clinical trials) the Patient Engagement Area is responsible.

We created a Young Person's Advisory Group (YPAG) in January 2015 with the aim to make the paediatric patients engagement in research feasible. KIDS Barcelona is the name of the group and it is formed by sixteen teenagers. They have been trained in four specific areas: biomedice, clinical research, innovation and clinical trials. All these areas are connected with the research projects that we perform in our organization.

In this paper we are going to share the most significant activities and projects that we have carried out with the involvement of the members of KIDS Barcelona. The examples have been selected with the aim to demonstrate that the active participation of young people in paediatric clinical research projects is feasible. It ensures that their needs are taken into account along all the processes of these projects.

Background about Patient Advocacy in Research

Huge experiences, more than 20 years, have demonstrated the benefits to involve adult patients in the field of research and clinical trials. Their contributions are positive for the projects in terms of return on investment (reducing time and costs) but above all in terms of return on engagement. This outcome is related to the opportunity to design clinical trials that can consider patient's particular needs and features, and this can have benefits to their quality of life.

Advocacy of adult patients or their representatives have experiences that cover all the different stages of clinical research (from the idetification of priorities to communicate the results of a study or to the dissemination of research findings). In the case of children the scenario is different, we have limited experiences and these are focused basically on the information addressed to young patients involved in clinical trials (patient information sheet and assent document).

The involvement of young advocates as active members of research projects has ethical concerns that we need to face, and due to the vulnerability of this population we need to respect their rights ensuring their privacy.

An ethical way to approach clinical research with young patients is through the forum of a Young Persons' Advisory Group. These are groups of young people interested in research, clinical trials, science and to become a young advocate for health research. Essential to their participation is that they receive the suitable training to ensure that they have the right knowledge and skills.

The leadership of these groups use to be a research centre or a patients' organization. This is positive to guarantee their privacy and to avoid any individual relationship with individuals that in this case are minors. In both cases they are directly connected with patients and the main goal of their activity is to increase the delivery of better research addressed to minors.

KIDS Barcelona: the YPAG of Sant Joan de Déu Children's Hospital

The group is led by the coordinator of the Clinical Research Unit and the coordinator of the Patient Engagement in Research Area. The team was created in January 2015 and is formed by sixteen teenagers (most of them patients) between 12 and 18 years old. In our country children above 12 years of age have to sign the assent document in order to demonstrate that they understand the scope of the research, the risks and benefits of their participation, and their rights, and that they voluntarily agree to take part in the clinical trial. For this reason we selected this age range, with the aim to ensure that the members of the group can deliver improvements in the documentation addressed to the patients that need to decide about their involvement in a clinical trial.

The option to involve healthy adolescents ensures that general questions or activities addressed to the members of the YPAGs are not going to have any disease bias.

The capacitation process of the members of KIDS Barcelona in the field of research lasted six months. The curriculum included content and skills about the four topics in which our hospital is performing projects: biomedicine, research, clinical trials and innovation. This educational content was performed by clinicians and researchers of our hospital, and had a practical approach about the different services related to these areas.

After the training process, the CEO of our Hospital welcomed the team as the Youth Scientific Council of the Hospital. This recognition makes feasible that the principal investigator of a project can ask for their consultation and advice. KIDS Barcelona members are part of the huge group of volunteers of our organization.

The meetings of KIDS Barcelona are held on a monthly basis and are led by two facilitators of the team. The methodology of every session follows a systematic process addressed to:
– Educate and empower the young people in the specific topic of the project for what is requested their participation. E.g. improve the assent document (language, content and format).
– Interactive activity to collect their feedback to improve the project using the best method to collect this information. E.g. focus groups, questionnaire, personal interviews, etc.

The content and the methods of the sessions are designed specifically for each project. In the first part of the session, the principal investigator of the project is the expert responsible to train the young people in the topic of the session. To offer them the background information of the project and the basis of the disease is essential in order to request their specific participation in the project. Afterwards, in the second part, the facilitators of the team perform practical activities to facilitate the process to discuss, deliberate and contribute to the project.

In the last three years the KIDS Barcelona team has been involved in several projects, among others these ones:

Case 1: Survey about the Children's and Adolescents' Views on Taking Medicines and Participating in Clinical Trials

The Paediatric Committee (PDCO) is the European Medicines Agency's (EMA) scientific committee responsible for activities on medicines for children and to support the development of such medicines in the European Union by providing scientific expertise and defining paediatric needs. PDCO prepared an easy survey with eleven questions targeting children and teenagers between 10 and 18 years of age. The questionnaire had two parts, one about the children's views on taking medicines (e.g. practical challenges such as palatability, formulation, etc.), and the second about their knowledge or experience with clinical trials. The survey was collected from March until May 2015 and the results are pending to be published by EMA.

The goal of this survey was to obtain information about preferences of this population related with pharmaceutical dosage and types, as well as the difficulties that one might face when consuming medicinal products. In addition, the goal was to elucidate their opinion about their possible involvement in research studies with drugs. Kids Barcelona members in collaboration with their educational institutions attained more than 500 answers.

This type of consultation is relevant. Usually the preferences of children are not questioned in the process to design a research project to study a new paediatric medicine. Hopefully this experience can be useful and be transferred to studies that might request the feedback of young patients along the design process.

Case 2: Feedback about Clinical Trials Addressed to Paediatric Patients

One of the areas in which young patient advocates can contribute, with adequate knowledge and capabilities, is the revision of clinical trial protocols. Members of Kids Barcelona have participated in the assessment of two protocols that we received from pharmaceutical companies, related to treatments addressed to Flu and Cystic fibrosis. Issues that were addressed and allowed the improvement of the initial study draft proposal included; palatability, frequency of medical appointments and follow-up visits, number of medical assessments, quality of life data, formulation preferences, and information for patients and families. Currently in collaboration with other groups, we are planning the development of a "guidance document" that will allow us to define the framework for collaboration with the pharmaceutical industry, research centres and regulators, which will unify standard procedures with the aim to standardize the approach of collaboration (types of consultation, methodologies, reporting, etc.) taking into consideration the particularities of this population.

Case 3: Launch of the European YPAG Network (eYPAGnet)

The European environment where paediatric clinical trials are performed requires the involvement of research centres from different countries. It is a key element to ensure the right recruitment of patients and to include the diversity in this process. If we are interested in increasing the involvement of young patients it is essential to have an infrastructure to connect the different YPAGs that already exist around Europe.

With the objective to setup a network of YPAGs and to promote the establishment of new ones, we created the eYPAGnet. This process was led by Generation R (UK), the ScotCRN (Scottish Children's Research Network), Kids France and Kids Barcelona. Together we represent the nine European groups that at the present moment exist.

In May 2017, eYPAGnet[1] achieved the accreditation of Enpr-EMA (European Networks of Paediatric Research of EMA) and was officially launched. During the next three years Hospital Sant Joan de Déu is going to coordinate the network on behalf of the team involved in KIDS Barcelona.

The goals of eYPAGnet are:
– Improve the capacity of collaboration with the different agents, who participate in the research process and development of innovative drugs.
– Gather a variety of experience related with different pathologies.
– Promote the planning and development of clinical research initiatives for children, on an European level.
– Consolidate the curriculum of capacity-building and empowerment training programs to the young patients.
– Promote and lead the creation of new groups.
– Empower the selection of professional careers in the scope of science, among the youth.

Case 4: Guidelines about the Content and Format of the Assent Document

Information provided to patients along the course of a clinical trial, is a particular challenge when the information is aimed at the paediatric population. In order to adapt the content to a suitable level of understanding KIDS Barcelona group created guidelines to recommend the adequate content and format of this important document. The outcome of their work was based on the analysis of 8 anonymous assent documents.

The guidelines include validation of ICAN (International Children's Advocacy Network) and EUPATI (European Patients on Therapeutic Innovation). It is available in Spanish[2] and English[3]. The document can be downloaded on the website of the Clinical Trials Unit of our hospital and in the Kids Barcelona website.

---

[1] European Medicines Agency (2017): *European Young Persons Advisory Groups Network*. URL http://bit.ly/eypagnet [10 November 2017].

[2] European Patients' Academy on Therapeutic Innovation (2017): *Consentimento informado en ensayos clínicos con pacientes pediátricos: el asentimiento. Recomendaciones para un diseño centrado en los niños.* URL http://bit.ly/asentimiento_pediatrico [10 November 2017].

[3] European Patients' Academy on Therapeutic Innovation (2017): *Informed consent document addressed to paediatric patients: the assent. Guidelines for a design focused on the children.*

This project was presented to the Ethics Committee of our organization and their members approved its content.

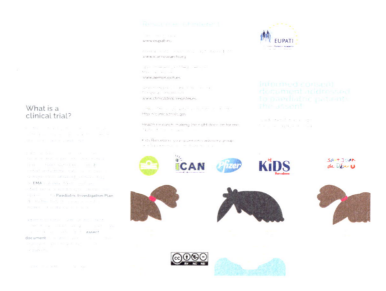

It was recently included in the instructions for the development of clinical trials with pediatric patients of the Spanish Regulatory Agency of Medicines and Medical Devices (AEMPS).[4]

The main recommendations that Kids Barcelona agreed to be considered in the design process of the assent document are:

Content	Format
– Concise content – Use vocabulary easy to understand – Include a general explanation of what a clinical trial is. – Easy understandable explanation of the possible side effects of the drug under study. – Include a glossary with definitions of the most difficult words to understand.	– Lenght from 2 to 5 pages. – Font size: between 12 and 14 points. – Always address the child in the second person singular. – Do not use the term "subject". – Use the term "patient" or "boy/girl". – Use colour, drawings, photos or infographics to facilite the comprehension of the information.

URL http://bit.ly/paediatric_assent [10 November 2017].

[4] Departamento de Medicamentos de Uso Humano (2016): *Guía para la correcta elaboración de un modelo de hoja de información al paciente y consentimiento informado (HIP/CI)*. URL http://bit.ly/aemps_asentimiento [10 November 2017].

If study sponsors take into consideration these recommendations in the process of designing the content and format of their consent/assent documents, we will contribute to ensure that the information will be understandable for the young patients. This needs to be the goal of this important and legal document. If we request the YPAGs' feedback to validate the content and format of the assent document, it can also contribute to ensure that the document fits its objective.

Case 5: Principles of Involvement of Patients in the Activities of European Medicines Agency

KIDS Barcelona, among the other founding members of eYPAGnet, was approached by the EMA to design the "**Principles on the involvement of patients in the activities of EMA**"[5].

The purpose of this framework is to establish rules for the involvement of young patients, consumers, and their carers, in the activities of the Agency's scientific committees and working parties in a consistent and efficient manner, whenever such involvement is appropriate in the interest of the ongoing scientific assessment within a particular (scientific) committee.

The main aims of the framework is to:[6]

– *Identify in which situations it may be helpful to seek input from young patients/consumers, their carers and the organisations they may be members of;*
– *Define what is expected from young patients/consumers/carers' involvement when they are consulted, and how best to capture their opinions;*
– *Establish an appropriate process to identify, support and consult with them.*

The involvement of eYPAGnet in the design of this framework ensures that the voice of the young people is included. The document "The role of patients as members of the EMA Human Scientific Committees"[7] was the starting point to develop this new framework. The main particularities regarding the needs of the young patients that can participate in the activities of EMA are:

– *Young patients/consumers and their carers should only be consulted in cases where their involvement can bring added value to the discussion, and it is for EMA/committee members/rapporteurs to decide on a case-by-case basis when it would be beneficial to consult them and the manner in which this consultation should take place.*

---

[5] European Medicines Agency (2017): *Principles on the involvement of young patients/consumers within EMA activities*. URL http://bit.ly/ema_framework [6 November 2017].
[6] European Medicines Agency (2017): *Principles on the involvement of young patients/consumers within EMA activities*. URL http://bit.ly/ema_framework [10 November 2017].
[7] European Medicines Agency (2011): *The role of patients as members of the EMA Human Scientific Committees*. URL http://bit.ly/ema_committees [10 November 2017].

- *The format of contact and dialogue for consultation needs to be agreed upon (for example, in person, via teleconference, in writing), and in addition necessary measures need to be in place to ensure that those participating do so in an appropriate manner.*
- *EMA can offer general and personalised support, and provide, including if possible a "mentor" speaking patient's own language to explain everything. This role can be performed by the facilitators of the YPAG.*

Examples where consultation/involvement could be of benefit during PDCO evaluation of Paediatric Investigation Plans:
- Proposed clinical trial design features (e.g. endpoints, randomisation, placebo, visit frequency, study duration, number of tests);
- Acceptability of route of administration, formulation, palatability, frequency of dosing, container systems and other packaging issues.
- Evaluations within COMP/PRAC/SAWP on specific paediatric medicines (pre & post-authorisation);
- Definition of therapeutic needs (not product specific), e.g. the development of guidelines.

These principles to involve young patients in the activities of a regulatory agency of medicines are the first around the world. It means that patient's voice can be considered during the assessment of the different stages addressed to achieve the marketing authorization of a new medicine.

Case 6: Collection of Educational Resources for Children and Young Patients about Clinical Research

Educational resources to explain the development of clinical trials are essential in order to help in the informative and consent process to paediatric patients. KIDS Barcelona has a huge expertise in the design of these resources that are used in the Clinical Research Unit of Sant Joan de Déu Children's Hospital and in other paediatric hospitals that collaborate with us in several projects.

The most relevant educational resources that we have developed are:
- **Video about what is a pediatric clinical trial**. The members of the YPAG designed the script and chose the cartoons of a short video that explains all the phases to perform a clinical trial addressed to children. The resource is accessible visiting this link: https://goo.gl/F2442G.
- **Video testimonial about the participation in a clinical trial**. Usually it is easy to understand an experience explained by people that have directly lived it. For this reason, we decided to participate in a video that gathers different testimonials (from children to adults) about the feelings and the experience of the involvement in a clinical trial. This resource can be useful for patients to compare their concerns with patient's that previously experienced the same

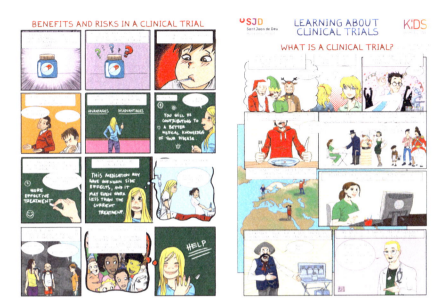

Two example pages of the comic about paediatric clinical trials.

challenging situation. The resource is accessible visiting this link: https://goo.gl/BpQ1ay.

- **Comic about the main concerns that young people have when they are participating in a clinical trial**. Explaining scientific concepts to young people is easier when we use the media and format that they use in their daily life. On the other hand, we need to consider that young patient's candidates to participate in a clinical trial are impacted by the burden of the disease and worried about the therapeutic options. This situation affects the information and consent process. For this reason, we decided that a comic would be an adequate resource to explain the main concerns that patients can have when they are asked to be involved in a clinical trial. We performed some interviews with patient's participating in clinical trials and we identified eight main concerns. Members of KIDS Barcelona chose the characters and prepared the script of the story. The resource allows two reading options: the whole story (across the eight topics) or only a single topic at a time (every page is addressed to cover one of the eight concerns). The topics covered are: what is a clinical trial, importance of clinical trials in children, phases of clinical trials, assent information, medical follow-up during the trial, benefits and risks, rights and "why me?". The resource is accessible visiting this link: https://we.tl/LaysXnVga1.

All the educational resources designed by the members of Kids Barcelona are available in Spanish and in English in the official website: www.kidsbarcelona.org.

Conclusions

YPAG is an ethical way of involving and engaging with young patients in the development of clinical trials, this ensures their rights and privacy. Groups include young people who have been trained in the field of clinical research and some of them having experience in the involvement of a clinical trial. They are not participating as individuals. This point can be a concern when we are involving minors.

Our experiences demonstrate that their participation along the process to perform a clinical trial is feasible. From the establishment of research priorities to the study design, from the creation of educational resources to the improvement of the content/format of the assent document. YPAGs can have a cross-cutting involvement to ensure that the voice and needs of the patients are taken into account in the whole drug development process.

The Ethical Principles Underpinning the Participation of Young People in the Development of Paediatric Clinical Research

Jennifer PRESTON, Pamela DICKS, Begonya Nafria ESCALERA,
Segolene GAILLARD

Introduction

The involvement of young people in research is an important ethical imperative[1] and has been called for by young people themselves.[2] 'Involvement' can be defined as when researchers collaborate with young people in the planning and management of studies to get patient input at all stages of the research process from the identification and priority of the research through to the dissemination of research findings in lay language.

Young people have historically been protected from medical research as some consider them as a vulnerable group that require protection, but recent arguments have shifted and advocates for young people's inclusion believe they have the right to the highest standards of health care, to be informed, express their views and influence decisions made about them.[3]

The valuable contribution that young people can make, both in paediatric study design, review and conduct of studies is increasingly being recognised. More importantly since 2009 and the introduction of the UN Convention of the Rights of the Child[4] there has been a move towards engaging young people directly in research, as opposed to relying on parents or carers to represent them, and a change in emphasis from research on children to research with children.[5] Reasons for young people's participation include, upholding their rights, fulfilling

---
[1] UNICEF (UK) (2010): *A Summary of the UN Convention on the Rights of the Child*, Article 36.
[2] Bate, J., Ranasinghe, N., Ling, R., Preston, J., Nightingale, R., Denegri, S. (2016): *Public and patient involvement in paediatric research*, in: Archives of Disease in Childhood – Education and Practice 0, 1–4. URL http://ep.bmj.com/content/early/2016/02/04/archdischild-2015-3095 00.extract [30 January 2018].
[3] Litt, I. F. (2003): *Research with, not on, adolescents: community-based participatory research*, in: The Journal of adolescent health 33 (5), 315–316.
[4] Franks, M. (2011): *Pockets of participation: revisiting child-centred participation research*, in: Children & Society 25 (1), 15–25.
[5] Sinclair, R., Franklin, A. (2000): *Young People's Participation*. Quality Protects Research Briefing No.3, London; Alderson, P. (2001): *Research by Children*, in: International Journal of Social Research Methodology 4 (2), 139–153; Kirby, P., Lanyon, C., Cronin, K., Sinclair, R. (2003):

legal responsibilities, improving services and decision-making, enhancing democratic processes, enhancing children's skills and empowering and enhancing self-esteem.[6]

The main aim of this chapter is to highlight the importance of involving young people in the design and development of paediatric clinical research. The chapter will also explore the challenges associated with involving young people effectively in this process and how the forum of a Young Person's Advisory Group can help in overcoming these challenges.

For the purpose of this chapter we refer to young people as those between the ages of eleven and eighteen years old who may have experience of a particular medical condition requiring medication, or who may not have a current illness but are able to represent the views and perspectives of young people more generally.

The Importance of Involving Young People

Although there is less of an evidence base in relation to young people's involvement in research practice than for adults, the case for their involvement has been explored in a number of publications.[7] Evidence suggests that by involving young people and their families it can lead to better research, clearer outcomes or more patient-focused outcomes and faster uptake of new evidence. Clinical trials that are more patient-focused are more likely to achieve required recruitment targets, and retain patients in the trial until completion. The benefits include, validity of the research, for example obtaining a better understanding of young people's worlds and health experiences or expectations; increased relevance and impact; benefits to those who get involved, for example skills, experience, recognition; and the ethics of involvement (rights, inclusion and empowerment). In order for involvement to be meaningful all these elements need to be in place. If there are no clear benefits to the research, and the ethics of involvement have not been considered then involvement is tokenistic. Furthermore, if there are no direct benefits to those involved then young people are unlikely to want to be, or stay, involved.

Building a Culture of Participation: involving children and young people in policy, service planning, delivery and evaluation, London; Staley K. (2009): *Exploring Impact: Public involvement in NHS, public health and social care research*, Eastleigh (UK).

[6] Hanley B., Bradburn, J., Barnes, M., Evans, C., Goodare, H., Kelson, M., Kent, A., Oliver, S., Thomas, S., Wallcraft, J. (2003): *Involving the Public in NHS, Public Health and Social Care Research: Briefing Notes for Researchers*, Second Edition, Eastleigh (UK); Kellett, M. (2005): *How to Develop Children as Researchers: a step by step guide to teaching the research process*, London.

[7] Hanley et al. 2003; Kellett 2005; Newman, J., Callens, C., Tibbins, C., Madge, N. (2012): *Medicines for Children. Reflecting on how young people improve research*, in: Fleming, J., Boeck, T. (eds.):Involving Children and Young People in Health and Social Care Research, New York, 165–174.

However, involving young people in the development of clinical research presents some challenges for those who design, conduct, monitor and participate in such activities. These challenges include, cultural differences and beliefs surrounding the involvement of young people; developing methodologies that encourage and enable young people to speak for themselves in their own ways, to be able to participate easily and to have their views interpreted meaningfully; organising meetings that suit young people's availability for example, during school holidays or weekends; ethical considerations regarding safeguarding and child protection and working with gatekeepers; having the available resources funding and expertise to facilitate active involvement, and having the ability to convince researchers of the importance of involving young people as partners in the research pathway.

Meaningful involvement needs to be planned from the outset and be properly resourced to include: discussions with young people in deciding if, when and how they want to be involved, and given all the information they need to do so in appropriate and accessible formats; involving young people in as many stages of process/project as possible and provide on-going support; be flexible and creative about models and methods of involvement, so that it is accessible and relevant to a wide range of young people; include elements over which young people have control, while being clear about the limits of autonomy; seek to find a balance between young people participation rights and ethical issues regarding safeguarding and child protection; consider appropriate methods of recognition; recruit, train, support and reward young people appropriately; ensure that all participation of young people in research activity is evidence-based, ethical, has clear benefits for young people involved as well as the researchers, and adheres to appropriate principles and best practices in relation to young people's participation; build in systematic evaluation of, and feedback on impacts and outcomes related to young people's involvement in research (for the individuals involved as well as for researchers and funders).

Involving Young People through the Forum of a Young Person's Advisory Group

One way to overcome these challenges is through the establishment of a Young Person's Advisory Group (YPAG) set up to empower young people and to influence different stages of the research pathway.

The first pilot YPAG was established in 2006 at Alder Hey Children's NHS Foundation Trust in the UK with support from the National Institute for Health Research (NIHR) Clinical Research Network (CRN): Children (what was then known as the Medicines for Children Research Network). The aim was to tackle the challenges mentioned above and to make sure young people were not placed in a predominantly adult environment where their contributions might be minimal. It was led by the principle that group activities should transform young people from research subjects into partners with researchers, with an active role and contribution to the projects.[8] Meetings were held at convenient times for group members (weekends or during school holidays) reimbursement of travel and subsistence to attend meetings was provided, as was a gift voucher as a thank you for contributing to group meetings. Learning and teaching activities were developed tapping into the creative/artistic/visual skills among the group, avoiding jargon and, most importantly, inviting researchers to the sessions so that young people could ask them about particular studies. Members of the group felt it was important if the researcher took the time and effort to speak to them directly. It also enabled young people to obtain written feedback from researchers as to what happened as a result of their input. For example, if they had suggested changes to a patient information leaflet, were their comments taken on board and how did the ethics committee regard these changes?

The pilot was a great success, which led to the establishment of a further five groups in England, and one in Scotland forming a national YPAG under the umbrella name of GenerationR (R for Research)[9]. Such groups were also established in France (KIDS France)[10] and Spain in 2015 (KIDS Barcelona).[11] At present twenty-four YPAGs exist in Europe, United States and Canada and numbers continue to grow.

The model of YPAGs is continuing to grow through the establishment of a virtual European YPAG Network (eYPAGnet) to support and promote the creation of YPAGs around Europe with the aim of giving more young people a voice at European level in the research process and to share best practices and learning between existing YPAGs. The main aim of eYPAGnet is to develop a centralized approach for the collaboration of YPAGs with the different working parties and committees of the European Medicines Agency (EMA)[12] including the Committee for Medic-

---

[8] Hanley et al. 2003; Kellett 2005.
[9] Wallace, E., Eustace, A. (2014): *Evaluation of Consumer Involvement in the NIHR Clinical Research Network: Children 2013-2014*, London. URL https://www.nihr.ac.uk/nihr-in-your-area/children/documents/CRN%20Children%20CI%20summary%20evaluation%20report%20January%202015%20copy.pdf [05 February 2018]; GenerationR (2018): *Young people improving health through research*. URL www.generationr.org.uk [30 January 2018].
[10] Le réseau d'Investigations Pédiatriques des Produits de Santé (ripps) (2018): URL www.ripps.eu [05 February 2018].
[11] KIDS Barcelona (2018): URL https://www.kidsbarcelona.org/en [05 February 2018].
[12] European Medicines Agency (2017): *Principles on the involvement of young patients/consumers within EMA activities*, EMA/494077/2016, 24 May 2017. URL http://www.ema.europa.eu/docs/en_GB/document_library/Regulatory_and_procedural_guideline/2017/07/WC500231645.pdf [05 February 2018].

inal Products for Human Use (CHMP) and the Paediatric Committee (PDCO) of the European Medicines Agency and to provide feedback to the scientific consultations that they receive from the research institutions and pharmaceutical companies. The eYPAGnet promotes the meaningful involvement of young people in European projects, allowing increased numbers of young advocates from different countries. This methodology also helps to include geographical and cultural differences existing between young people around Europe.

On of the main goals of eYPAGnet includes designing a common curriculum that educates, informs and equips YPAGs with the knowledge of drug development and discovery, as well as focusing on the ethical aspects of undertaking health research with young people. This teaching has formed a major part of the activities already undertaken with well established YPAGs and includes ethical debates such as: benefits and risks involved in participating in research; at what age should young people be able to decide to take part in research; should young people be allowed to have the final say to participate; what happens if a young person decides they no longer want to be in a study and is the information given to them age appropriate to ensure fully informed consent or assent. The latter point has been a major issue for a number of years and YPAGs continue to receive study information that is too long, complicated, sometimes patronizing and important information lost through the use of too much science. The ethos behind involving young people in reviewing such information is that this will lead to the production of more child-appropriate information that young people feel empowered to read and make their own decisions to participate in important decision, obviously with support from their families.

To overcome this issue eYPAGnet have recently worked in partnership with the Ethics Working Group of Enpr-EMA to develop a standardized template of the consent/assent document. This involved activities that included: an introduction of an assent template proposed by the Working Group; reading and discussion about its main features, and collection of individual feedback of all the attendees through a questionnaire that included open ended questions about what was important and less important information that should be included in the patient information sheet. Discussions around how much information is too much, what format should it be in and in what order also took place. In summary feedback from the sessions included young people wanting information sheets to be more practical to include and focus more attention on what treatments young people are likely to receive as part of the research, which is different to what they would normally receive as part of routine care; likely side-effects of the treatment; how long will they be in the study; how will taking part in the research affect my life, for example impact on school work and social life; information about contraception and alcohol use and where to find additional information. Information young people did not think was necessary was who funds the research and the explanation of ethical approval. In terms of how the information should be presented the groups felt that the layout should be clear with short blocks of texts; inclusion of bullet points; tables are good to summarise text; photos and diagrams are helpful if relevant to the text; a glossary might help; charts showing visits and length of stay and a list of additional resources to read more information if they wish to should be provided. Most importantly young people felt that all patient information sheets aimed at young people should be approved by them to ensure that it meets their needs and will aid the decision to participate in research. Ethics committees should consider this for all paediatric studies where appropriate.

Feedback from this exercise was forwarded to Enpr-EMA Working Group to be carefully reviewed against the new 'Pediatric Ethics Guideline' together with comments from the European Academy of Pediatrics and will be made publicly available on the Enpr-EMA website when finalized. In turn this will ultimately assist researchers to prepare information that is fit for purpose and aid the decision making process for young people invited to participate in clinical trials.

Conclusion

Since the adoption of the United Nations Convention on the Rights of the Child (UNCRC) the ethos to involve and engage young people in the decision-making process of peadiatric clinical trials has increased, and has been witnessed in the growth of YPAGs across the Globe. The formation of YPAGs has enabled young people to become more involved in the research process by giving them the confidence, information and opportunities to be able to contribute at all levels. Age appropriate information, and trial design that considers the specific requirements of young people improves communication with young people and thereby facilitates consent and assent and recruitment to clinical trials.

However, to achieve the greatest benefit from the involvement of young people, participation should be integral to the entire process from the outset and the establishment of a European YPAG network is one way to achieve this aim. The network will work hard to strengthen collaborations and partnerships with members of the EMA to ensure young people have a voice throughout the entire research pathway. We will continue to provide support to anyone who wishes to effectively involve and engage young people in clinical research, educate young people about drug discovery and development and more importantly develop the tools to build on the evidence base of the impact of young people involvement in the design and delivery of paediatric clinical research. This is just the beginning and we have a long way to go to ensure all young people regardless of their cultural, ethnic, religious backgrounds have the opportunities to have their say on matters that concern them.

Young People, Deliberation, and Research Ethics: A Film Project by the Nuffield Council on Bioethics

Kate HARVEY

Introduction

In May 2015, the Nuffield Council on Bioethics[1] launched a report which examined ethical issues associated with children's and young people's involvement in clinical research.[2] To inform the report's conclusions, a range of engagement activities with young people were undertaken throughout the two-year project, including the formation of a stakeholder group of young people to advise the project team; devising an animated film with the guidance of young people; and working with young people when preparing drafts of the written report and accompanying materials.[3]

In addition to these engagement activities, a film initiative launched at the beginning of the two-year project sought to compare young people's and adults' responses to ethical issues raised by a fictional research protocol. This chapter will focus on the film project's aims, methods, and conclusions.

Background

In order for the project to capture as many perspectives pertinent to paediatric health research as possible, it was imperative that children and young people were involved meaningfully throughout the course of the Council's work. In some of the engagement activities which supported this project, the views and input of young people with *direct* experience of clinical research were actively sought, and provided valuable insights and contributions to the project.[4]

---

[1] Nuffield Council on Bioethics (2018): *Exploring ethical issues in biology and medicine.* URL http://nuffieldbioethics.org/ [01 March 2018]. The Council is an independent organisation which was established in 1994. It has achieved an international reputation for advising policy-makers and stimulating debate in bioethics.

[2] Nuffield Council on Bioethics (2015): *Children and clinical research: ethical issues*, London, UK. URL http://nuffieldbioethics.org/wp-content/uploads/Children-and-clinical-research-full-report.pdf[01 March 2018].

[3] For further information on the Council's engagement with young people for this project, see Appendices 2, 3, 4, and 5 of the report.

[4] These included the participation and input of young people in a stakeholder group established for the course of the project, and members of young persons' advisory groups (YPAGs) across the UK (see paragraph 3.38 of the report for further information on the work of YPAGs).

However, when a young person finds himself / herself in a scenario where clinical research participation is offered to them, they may often not have knowledge of what clinical research 'is' and how it 'works'. It was therefore imperative to consider the perspective of young people *without* direct experience of clinical research in considering ethical issues in this context. This group's views were considered and captured through filmed group discussions that resulted in a series of videos which are now freely and publicly available.[5]

The film project took as its inspiration the discussions held by research ethics committees (RECs) to assess the ethical acceptability of a clinical research protocol. It was split into two parts which will hereafter be referred to as 'Adult REC' and 'Youth REC', each part of which is explained in the method section below.

Ethics approval for the project was granted by the Institute of Education at the University of London. The co-application was submitted by the Nuffield Council, and three supporting academic researchers.

Aims of the Film Project

The general aims of the film project were:

To consider young people's views of ethical issues raised by a fictional (but true-to-life) research protocol;

To identify areas of consensus and disagreement between adults and young people when they are asked to consider the same research protocol;

To inform future approaches to research ethics training and education;[6] *and*

To give paediatric clinical researchers and the RECs who consider their research protocols an opportunity to reflect on and observe young people's ability to consider and assess complex research protocols.

---

[5] In addition to the two films which are explored at length in this chapter, a further short film which provides a 'trailer' gives an introduction to the film project and the themes which emerged from it. URL http://nuffieldbioethics.org/project/children-research/films-young-peoples-perspectives-clinical-ethics-reviews [01 March 2018].

[6] Following the completion of the film project, the Nuffield Council published a set of educational resources to support this aim. These included a flexible workshop plan for use with a group of young people which sets out different activity options that use the films, such as a role play exercise, and a group discussion. URL http://nuffieldbioethics.org/wp-content/uploads/Research Ethics_plan.pdf [01 March 2018].

Method

Development of a Fictional Research Protocol

Prior to the commencement of filming, a fictional research protocol was developed. While fictional, every care was taken to ensure that the protocol – which focused on a novel way of identifying the most appropriate treatment for childhood asthma, given children's variable responses to two standard medications – *could* be genuine. To achieve this, advice was sought from a consultant / clinical researcher in paediatric asthma care in developing the fictional protocol.[7] The protocol itself was designed to prompt responses from the Adult REC and Youth REC on particular ethical points, such as consent, risk, and privacy.

The fictional protocol[8] – titled *Asthma treatments for children with the MAS gene: a clinical trial assessing the efficacy of Exhalin vs Verabreath*[9] – proposed to change the way that children with severe asthma are assigned their 'stage 3' medication. (Stage 1 and stage 2 medication involve the use of blue (reliever) and brown (preventer) inhaler, respectively; stage 3 medications are tablets taken orally.) The protocol was based on the theory that children with a particular gene (referred to as the 'MAS gene') may not react well to the standard prescription they receive for their stage 3 medication (Exhalin), and that this group may therefore react better to Verabreath.

The protocol suggested splitting 200 children aged 7-18 into two equal groups. The 100 participants in the first group would have their saliva tested to see if they have the MAS gene: if they did, they would be given Verabreath in addition to their blue and brown inhalers (group 1a). If they did not, then they would continue to take the standard stage 3 treatment (Exhalin) (group 1b). Group 2 participants would not have their saliva tested for the MAS gene, and would be treated on a 'trial and error' basis (i.e. the standard approach clinicians take to identifying the best course of treatment for a particular patient).

Outcomes for participants in groups 1 and 2 would then be compared, with reference to analysing school attendance and using an online survey to assess the frequency with which the participants used their blue inhaler for the duration of the trial (one year). Overall, the protocol aimed to observe whether aggregated outcome measures in the genotype-directed prescribing model (group 1) are better than those reached by the usual 'trial and error' model (group 2).

---

[7] Professor Somnath Mukhopadhyay, Brighton and Sussex Medical School. URL https://www.bsms.ac.uk/about/contact-us/staff/professor-somnath-mukhopadhyay.aspx[01 March 2018].

[8] A full account of the study in the form of an application for ethics approval is available online: Nuffield Council on Bioethics (2018): *Improving asthma treatments for children and young people. Application for ethics approval*. URL http://nuffieldbioethics.org/wp-content/uploads/Mock-application-asthma-treatments-study1.pdf[01 March 2018].

[9] Both the drug names 'Exhalin' and 'Verabreath', and the 'MAS' gene are fictional.

The fictional protocol was designed to include several ethical issues / points of debate. For example:

Participants may already know the researcher who is leading the project, as he is the doctor for some of them.

Participants can only take part if their parents give permission, regardless of age. If their parents refuse permission, the young person will not be able to participate.

Participants' general practitioners will be contacted as standard to make them aware of the details of the study.

The protocol refers to 'research subjects' rather than 'research participants'.

The protocol requires participants to discontinue their current stage 3 medication for a period of two-weeks before the research begins to 'wash out' the effects of their standard medication, and to avoid compounding factors in the research. (i.e., participants can use only their inhalers, and not additional tablets, for a period of two weeks ahead of the study.) This could potentially cause discomfort or distress to participants and also bring about opportunity costs such as being unable to play sport.

Some participants will be tested to see if they have the MAS gene. DNA (saliva) samples will be kept by the researchers for (undefined) "future research questions".

One of the outcome measures of the fictional protocol is to assess the number of absence days recorded on participants' school registers. Permission will be sought from participants' parents and their schools to obtain these data.

A second outcome measure will require participants to complete a confidential online survey to establish the frequency with which participants in each group use their inhalers while taking part in the study (comparing the use of inhalers between each group).

Participants will be asked to spend a half-day in hospital four times during the one-year research period. They will be asked to have a number of tests, including for testing their lung function and how they cope with exercise. The results of these tests will be matched against the self-reported information obtained via the online surveys, and participants' attendance records.

The research findings will be published in a publicly-accessible document. One of the researchers will also use the results of the study to complete his PhD.

Participants will receive a £20 voucher to thank them for their participation. Travel expenses for participants and their parents / guardians will be reimbursed by the research team.

Some of these issues were commented on explicitly by both Adult and Youth RECs; others were highlighted more strongly by one REC but not the other; whereas some ethical issues were not drawn out by either group. The focus, or lack of, on these issues by both adult and youth groups is explored in detail in the **key themes** section below.

Adult REC Preparation and Filming

The Adult REC was comprised of six individuals with experience of ethics committee deliberations.

Taking the fictional research protocol as its basis, a series of other materials were developed to present to the Adult REC for consideration. The distributed materials were:[10]

- Application for ethics review (used as the basis for the meeting's agenda)
- Covering letter for parents and guardians
- Information sheet for parents and guardians
- Consent form for parents and guardians
- Information sheet for children and young people (potential participants)
- Assent form for children and young people (potential participants)

Over the course of an hour, the assembled Adult REC members were invited by the REC Chair to highlight their initial thoughts or ethical concerns about the protocol and its materials. Following discussions of the protocol, Adult REC members were then asked by the Chair to come to a decision about the protocol: whether it should be approved as presented; or if there were requirements that needed to be fulfilled for approval.

All of the Adult REC's discussions were filmed by a documentary filmmaker[11], and were subsequently edited as a contributory element of 16-minute film titled *Processes, papers and professors: how clinical research in young people gets approved* (hereafter 'Film One')[12].

Film One: Narrative and Content

The purpose of Film One was to construct a prompt for discussions which would contribute to a second film (see **Youth REC participation and filming** below), and to give background information on the protocol being examined.

In addition to presenting the Adult REC's discussions, Film One introduced a seven-year-old girl called Ruby, who lives with severe asthma and is a patient of the consultant who advised the Council on the development of the protocol. The involvement of Ruby was paramount in enabling a narrative to thread throughout both films and to enliven the presentation of ethics committee discussions. Ruby's and her family's consent was documented in advance of filming.

---

[10] These materials are available on request from the Nuffield Council.
[11] Vivianne Howard, Creative Director, Helter Skelter Studios. URL http://helterskelterstudios.com/creative-director/ [01 March 2018].
[12] Film One is available online: Nuffield Council on Bioethics (2014): *Processes, Papers and Professors: how clinical research in young people gets approved*. URL https://www.youtube.com/watch?v=VaiZ58uiwdU [01 March 2018].

The filmmaker edited Film One into six scenes:
- **Scene 1**: Background information on the protocol, through the introduction of Ruby and her family. The consultant / researcher also appears in this scene to comment further on the severity of Ruby's asthma. The viewer is invited to take into account the effects of asthma on Ruby's life, including her medicines routine.
- **Scene 2**: This scene takes places in a children's hospital in Brighton, a city on the south coast of the UK (and the hospital that Ruby attends for her consultations with her consultant). It sees Ruby preparing to meet her consultant to discuss her treatment.
- **Scene 3**: The consultant explains the hypothesis of the fictional protocol he has sent to the Adult REC for discussion.
- **Scene 4**: This scene further establishes the details of the protocol which the consultant sent to the Adult REC for discussion. It also introduces to the viewer, in simple terms, the function of an ethics committee.
- **Scene 5**: The Adult REC discusses the protocol and its associated ethical issues at length. Each member sets out their concerns with the terms of the protocol, and how those concerns might be addressed by the researcher. The scene ends with the Chair closing the meeting and indicating the committee's intention to write a letter to the researcher to ask for aspects of the protocol to be re-examined or re-designed.
- **Scene 6**: The consultant / researcher awaits the arrival of an email from the Adult REC regarding whether the protocol has been approved, or needs to be amended. The researcher receives the Adult REC's decision and responds to some of their concerns. For example: "they are not very pleased with us referring to the children as 'subjects' rather than 'participants', and I think that this is a very valid point." The scene, and the film, ends with an emphasis on the importance of young people's participation in clinical research.

Youth REC Preparation and Filming

On the completion of Film One, the next stage of the project commenced. This stage involved engaging with young people across three different schools in Brighton. The young people involved in this part of the study were students at a junior school, secondary school, and sixth form college (at ages 10-11, 12-16, and 16-18, respectively). The three schools were selected to include a broad spectrum of socioeconomic locations.

Each school was asked to identify 6-8 students who might be asked to take part in filming a second piece and be confident enough to speak in front of a camera. Once participants were identified and consent for filming was obtained from participants and their parents, three one-day filming workshops were arranged to take place at each of the participating schools. Each filming workshop lasted approximately two hours. The structure of the Youth REC workshops is set out in **Box 1** below.[13]

Box 1: Structure of Mock Youth REC Workshops

1. Warm-up activity on participants' views on what is meant by 'clinical research' and 'research ethics'.
2. Viewing scenes 1-4 of Film One (Part I), to help participants to understand why clinical research might be important.
3. Facilitated discussion with participants to encourage debate around key concerns and ethical issues associated with the mock research protocol and its associated materials (information sheets, assent / consent forms, and explanatory letters to parents of potential mock research participants).
4. Viewing scenes 5-6 of Film One (Part II).
5. Facilitated discussion to explore what the Youth RECs thought of the adults' conclusions, drawing out similarities and differences with their own thoughts.

Students who participated in the workshops did not receive copies of the research protocol and its associated materials in advance of filming. Instead, an academic researcher with extensive experience of facilitating qualitative research with young people led each workshop and discussed explanatory materials with the Youth REC, including a background information sheet on what 'research ethics' means and, in addition to the same protocol that the Adult REC considered, a separate information sheet on the fictional trial explaining *'what's it all about?'*.

Subsequently, participants were invited to set out what ethical issues they could identify with the protocol. They were also shown Film One in two parts: scenes 1-4 comprised Part I; scenes 5-6 comprised Part II. The purpose of screening Film One in two parts was to ensure that the young people's views on the protocol were not influenced by the Adult REC's conclusions. However, the participants were given an opportunity to discuss the Adult REC's conclusions *after* they had reached their own. This approach enabled clear comparisons to be drawn

---

[13] See further: Nuffield Council on Bioethics (2014):*"What we think about what adults think"*. *Children and young people's perspectives on ethics review of clinical research with children*. URL http://nuffieldbioethics.org/wp-content/uploads/Report_young_peoples_perspectives_on_ethics_review.pdf[01 March 2018].

between the adults' and young people's conclusions on the ethical aspects of the fictional protocol.

All of the young people's discussions were filmed by the same documentary filmmaker who had worked with the project team on the Adult REC's discussions.

Film Two: 'Be a part of it: What Young People Think of Clinical Research'[14]

Once the three school workshops were complete, the filmmaker edited a second film that presented the young people's discussions and reintroduced particular parts of the Adult REC's discussions. The film was edited this way in order to show that the young people's concerns both mirrored and, in some cases, contradicted those of the Adult REC in several respects. The structure of Film Two is set out in **Box 2** below.

Box 2: structure of Film Two

Establishes the aim of the project (i.e., to learn what young people think about the research studies adults devise and the decisions they make about children's involvement in clinical research).

Sets out what young people think 'ethics' means.

Notes that the film will seek to establish young people's views of what ethical issues apply to the protocol on asthma that has been presented to them at the workshops.

Provides a brief recap of the purpose of the study (i.e., to establish whether there is a better way of treating childhood asthma, based on treating according to the presence of the MAS gene).

Introduces the Adult REC and the tasks of a REC in clinical research contexts. The young people are then asked to 'become' a REC and to discuss the protocol in the same way that Adult RECs do.

The majority of Film Two, however, focuses on **key themes** raised by the young people in response to the fictional research protocol. Each of these themes is explored in full in the next section of this chapter, which draws comparisons between the Youth REC's and Adult REC's conclusions on each key theme.[15]

---

[14] Nuffield Council on Bioethics (2014): *Be a part of it: What Young People Think of Clinical Research*. URL https://www.youtube.com/watch?v=e2k6eA0dn9Q [01 March 2018].

[15] This analysis relates only to the discussions which appear in Films One and Two. Other discussions of Adult and Youth REC members that were not edited into the final film versions are not included.

A Film Project by the Nuffield Council on Bioethics

Key Themes of the Youth REC's Discussions: Comparisons With the Adult REC

A Personal Approach to Research Participants

Youth REC members strongly emphasised the need for researchers to take a personal approach to their potential research participants.

One of the Youth REC's specific points focused on the lack of apparent forethought by the researchers regarding how their protocol could affect research participants, and their families. One Youth REC member criticised the researchers, observing, "I don't think they have actually thought about the children in this situation, or how it can affect the adults [i.e., parents and guardians] as well." Another young person observed that the researchers "shouldn't think of all the participants as a whole group of people but more as individuals, because everyone has different lives and it could affect them in different ways." Other comments by the Youth REC which echo this view included:

"The researchers need to think about the children in this situation because it could really affect these children's benefits and their future."

"They just need to make sure that they consider all the young people's feelings – what they might be thinking."

Youth REC participants also highlighted the importance of building relationships in order to create a personalised approach to clinical research. For example, one Youth REC member suggested that researchers "should work really closely with the [participants'] doctors so that they know the children more and they have a close relationship", and another emphasised the importance of forging a "personal connection between the researcher and the participants" so that "the study is as personal as it can be". Another suggestion by Youth REC members included:

"I think it would be important to make sure that they are actually realising that it is the children that are taking part in it and not the parents. So make all the consent forms and information sheets relevant to the children and then maybe give out different ones to the parents and then they can decide which one fits their child the best."

The Adult REC also highlighted their concerns regarding a 'personal' approach through flagging the researchers' use of the term 'research subject' rather than 'research participant' in their application form and information sheets. The Adult REC's concerns about the message conveyed by the use of 'subject' rather than 'participant' was further noted in the Nuffield Council's subsequent report, which observes: "Clinical research must always be with children and young people, not 'on' them: they are not mere passive subjects but rather active participants in a joint enterprise of research."[16]

Clarity of Communication

Youth REC members highlighted several aspects of the protocol that they felt lacked clarity of communication from the researchers.

Language

The language used in the documents presented by the researchers to the Youth REC was criticised for being too complicated. One Youth REC member stated that "some of the language, particularly on this sheet – for lots of children that would go straight over their heads. They would need a conversation with the doctor of what's it about."

Similarly, the Adult REC highlighted the age range that the research protocol proposed to include (7-18), but noted that the written information provided would be too complicated for younger participants, and also too patronising for older participants. As a result, the Adult REC was left with the impression that the research team did not 'understand' children and young people.

The protocol design and details

The research team were further criticised for failing to provide sufficient details on key aspects of the fictional protocol. One Youth REC participant noted especially the need for the researcher to better explain how they would test the outcomes of their trial:

"In the consent form they don't really explain properly how they are going to test the outcomes of it and sometimes young people don't know exactly what all these tests are called and they've used the proper healthcare names for them. But it needs to be something that is properly explained and how often they are going to have to do that."

The Adult REC highlighted safety concerns around the protocol's design. For example, they noted that it is unclear whether the control group will have their care and treatment compromised by their participation in the study. The Youth REC also noted that it is important to know "if there was any research behind the safety of a washout period and how that would physically affect children." The researcher acknowledges this point in Film Two, and notes that the research on

---

[16] Nuffield Council on Bioethics 2015, paragraph 80.

washout periods for this type of asthma medication could be set-out more clearly in his protocol.

The Adult REC also urged the researchers to reconsider their outcome measures, and to include other measures, such as the frequency with which participants use their reliever medication while participating in the trial; and what their peak flow measurement is.[17]

Alternative means of communication

The Youth REC proactively suggested ways through which the researchers might improve the quality of their communication, particularly the potential use of other formats such as video.

"Maybe show something that explains it, so people show you a video or clip. That could explain it."

"If there are a lot of children that could be taking part, it could be quicker for them to get the information. The GP could just give them a DVD or a website to go and look at it."

"I think there should be both an information sheet and a video."

The Adult REC did not highlight the potential of alternative formats in their discussion.

Engaging with Participants and Families

Participants in Youth REC discussions indicated that the researchers who devised the fictional protocol should aim to engage meaningfully with their potential participants. One Youth REC member suggested: "maybe the person in charge of the experiment could come in and talk to the children and explain what it really is about." This suggestion links clearly with **point (1)** above and the participants' emphasis on adopting a personal approach to clinical research.

The Adult REC highlighted a complementary point: it observed that the research team had omitted to speak to young people "upfront" and clarify what was important to them in their role of potential research participants. They felt that it was crucial to involve potential participants from the outset so that concerns around participants being treated as subjects of research, rather than research participants, could be allayed.

The Adult REC also suggested that if young people who were allowed to be part of the *development* of the research study, it would be more likely that they

---

[17] For general information on the peak flow test, see: NHS choices (2018): *Peak flow test*. URL https://www.nhs.uk/conditions/peak-flow-test/ [01 March 2018].

understand the whole research process. The Adult REC similarly observed that initial consent to participate in the study should not be the end of children's and parents' / guardians' involvement: rather, they should be engaged *throughout* the project.

Youth REC members also emphasised that the researchers should engage with participants' family members. Their reasons for indicating the importance of this included:

"It could lead to dangerous outcomes that the parents may not know how to handle – so if they were just ill in the night and they didn't know how to handle it they would have to go to the hospital."

"The doctors should tell the children what it's all about and what could be the possible effects to it and definitely tell the adults – the parents – what they might be going through, what will happen."

The Adult REC also felt that the researchers had provided parents with insufficient information on the risk of their child's participation, particularly in respect of safety concerns around the washout period specified by the protocol. The Adult REC asked: "Whom should they [parents] contact? Where do they get advice from?"

Consent: Involving Parents and Guardians

The Adult REC and Youth REC came to quite different conclusions on the role of parents and guardians in giving consent to research participation.

The Adult REC firmly noted that some of the potential participants would be old enough to have children and vote and that, therefore, the requirement that only parents could consent to their participation was not appropriate. However, Youth REC members – at both ends of the age spectrum – uniformly stated that they would expect their parents to help them to make decisions to take part in clinical research; and, moreover, would *welcome* their views and advice.

"Personally if my parents told me I wasn't allowed to take part in the trial, I think that I would listen to them cos I would kind of trust their judgment on whether they think it was safe or not." [Participant in the 16-18 age bracket]

The workshops also highlighted that children in the younger age brackets wanted to be actively involved in research participation decisions.

"My brother's eight and I know that he would like to have a say with probably my mum and dad."

"I think it should be a joint decision but it also depends on how old you are, like, say you are 10, like me, I would want to have a say but my parents decide with me because they

might know what's better and what the test is all about and I might not be as bothered as they are."

"I would like to have my say but my parents to help me out with it . . . "

Balancing Risk, Burden and Benefit

Both the Youth REC and Adult REC criticised the information provided around the risks, burdens, and benefits of the study. The Adult REC suggested strongly that the risks and potential benefits of the research should be set out more clearly, a view echoed by several Youth REC members:

"They should be told first of all what could go wrong and if they are still willing to do it, they should be able to do it. If they know that it might be painful and they still want to go through with it, then I don't really see anything wrong with that. But like if they are just told 'we are going to do some research on you, this is what we are going to do but don't say anything but it could go wrong' – then, that's bad!"

"And also if it turns out that the medicine didn't work on them and they weren't on the other things [drugs] which were helping then they're pretty much in a bad situation cos they will be putting them that much more at risk."

"He said he would have to leave a child without medication for two weeks and if he is only testing people with serious asthma and if you had serious asthma – two weeks – you could have an asthma attack in two weeks if you didn't have any medication at all."

"If you just leave them without it they're going to be having asthma attacks and they are going to be ill and they're going to get infections in the lungs and stuff."

" . . . also if it could go wrong how they [the researchers] would deal with it."

The Adult REC also highlighted specifically whether it is acceptable to stop the third line defence medication of children with serious asthma, and asked whether it might be preferable to invite children to take part in the research at the point at which they begin taking their third line drug.

One Youth REC member, however, suggested that drawing attention to the risks of the protocol could affect recruitment: "If they tell you – you are going to have loads of side effects and stuff like that you're probably not going to really want to do it."

Potential burdens that might arise for participants who agree to take part in the trial were also highlighted by Youth REC members. Again, they felt that the researchers had not given sufficient thought to the ways that participating in the research might affect participants' wider interests.

"I think it is important to consider not only the health effect but actually the effect on the child's day to day life and how that will physically affect them and how many times they would have to go up to hospital."

"Well it's quite like it's taking away your freedom, if you have to always do tests like every week or something then you won't have much time to do what you actually want to in your normal life."

"The tests can make you really exhausted and all these things that you do on you so you get back home and you're really exhausted so you won't be able to do as much things, just sleep all the time."

When referring to outcome measures, the Adult REC similarly highlighted the burdens that might beset research participants, such as not being able to take part in sports or social activities.

Youth REC members also noted the omission of reference to the potential *benefits* of taking part in this piece of research.

"If you only had to take one or two tablets instead of a lot then it would make morning routines quicker and easier."

"Maybe in the future we're able to help to cure asthma and to stop asthma attacks."

Concerns around Privacy, Confidentiality, and Data Management

Youth REC members expressed significant concern about the researchers' approach to privacy, confidentiality, and data management. Some Youth REC members also expressed explicit concern about the researchers' motives for gathering and storing their data.

"They're too personal though… When they're asking you your postcode [zip code], it's so obvious it's not anonymous."

"When people say this person won't say anything around people, like they are saying if you have ever done drugs, if you ever smoked, if you ever had alcohol. So they know and they are asking for your postcode – it's pretty obvious that they are going to be sending this information off if you say the wrong thing like you do drugs or you smoke or you've ever had alcohol before."

"This information could go anywhere. It could go to people that are going to make something out of it, it could go to people who are going to do something bad with it. It could go to good causes and stuff. You know what it's about but you don't know how it is going to be used."

"It's the government. Well the government never keeps their promises."

"Seven year olds might not understand but later in life it could be used against them somehow."

"You might want to find out who's going to be looking at all of this cos it might be like, say, universities or it could be like just people you know and that might affect whether you want to do it or not."

"I was quite shocked that they didn't put the DNA thing in the consent form cos that's quite important – and also what would happen to the DNA after the study taking place… ?"

"It could be quite invasive if they have to continually answer questions about their life."

The Adult REC raised similar concerns about the future use of saliva samples that the researchers proposed to take as part of the study, and the fact that no information was provided on its future use. This omission of further information on the protocol and the accompanying consent forms was, they suggested, "remarkable".

Information about 'what happens' once the Research Ends

Among Youth REC members, there was also a desire for more information on what the results of the study would contribute to once the research ended, and also, more broadly, 'what happens next' to research participants. Conversely, the Adult REC did not raise this issue in its discussions.

"It wouldn't be good if they were doing it for no reason at all… it is good if you know what's actually happening to the results and why they're doing it."

"For me they have to make sure they consider what happens once they have finished their study and make sure that the drugs they are giving and all the treatments they are giving are sustainable. You don't want to give them a drug that makes them feel loads better and then just suddenly pull it from beneath them."

Incentives, Rewards, and Altruism

Members of the Adult REC did not agree regarding whether the proposal to give a £20 voucher to research participants was appropriate. One of the adults felt that it was a patronising amount to give participants, and that it was "not a lot of money". However, another Adult REC member argued that children's altruistic motives for research participation should not be underestimated, and that a £20 voucher was a sufficient gesture; "a cherry on top of the cake". The same member suggests that more worry would result if participants were to be given too *much* money.

Among Youth REC members, similar disagreements occurred on the appropriateness of the gift voucher. Some of the young people on the Youth REC questioned, for example, whether the relatively low monetary value of the voucher undermined whether the research was 'worth' doing.

"If I was 7 or 8 I would probably want to do it for an Amazon voucher but now that I am older I'd probably be, like, it is it worth it?"

Other Youth REC participants, however, felt that the voucher represented a bribe.

"I think that it is kind of a bit of a bribe, that maybe the children might be – I don't know – they could be swayed into thinking one certain thing if they were getting a treat out of it."

"If they don't really want to do it and you get loads of stuff afterwards – well it's kind of bribing them to do it."

One young person also recommended an alternative to a voucher with a clear monetary value attached, instead suggesting "if they were going to give a reward it should be like a day out with the family or something that they know that the children would enjoy as well."

Youth REC members also put forward a strong argument around the importance of altruism (rather than monetary incentives) to participate in research.

"I don't think they should get money at all because it's helping other children for finding different cures and you don't have to be paid to be a nice person, do you? … You get to choose if you want to do that and you don't get paid for being a good person."

"I think that people should do it out of the goodness of their hearts rather than for the money. Because that means if they are risking their lives to help everyone in the future rather than just helping themselves, it would be much more selfless! If you don't want to do it then that is fine too – cos you don't want to die. But if you do it – it's doing it out of the goodness of your heart."

"In my opinion I actually think I would do it if I had asthma – I would. I wouldn't do it for any money, any vouchers – nothing. I would just do it cos it is helping myself, I might find a cure, but it is actually helping other people with bad asthma. It could change the world."

Conclusions

The films highlight that young people are more than capable of considering the same research protocol as a group of adults, provided that the protocol is appropriately presented (for example, through summarising key points of the protocol in age-appropriate language, or facilitating discussions with young people in an accessible, inclusive way).

The film project showed that although some points of note and concern were mirrored in adults' and children's consideration of the protocol, their views differed in key areas (for example, around consent and incentives). The young people also raised new points that the Adult REC had not considered, such as the importance of clarity around 'what happens' at the conclusion of the research trial. The contribution of young people to the research ethics approval process is therefore an addition that can therefore potentially add context to, and personalise, research, as well as providing researchers with new ideas and perspectives that add to the integrity of their studies.

Medizin-Ethik / Medical Ethics
Schriftenreihe des Arbeitskreises Medizinischer Ethik-Kommissionen in Deutschland
hrsg. von Dirk Lanzerath
in Verbindung mit
Joerg Hasford und Sebastian Graf von Kielmansegg

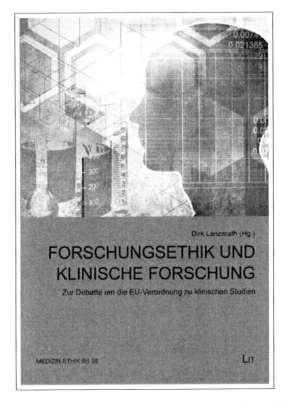

Dirk Lanzerath (Hg.), in Verbindung mit dem Vorstand des AK der medizinischen Ethikkommissionen
Forschungsethik und klinische Forschung
Zur Debatte um die EU-Verordnung zu klinischen Studien
Die neue EU-Verordnung für die Neuregelung der klinischen Prüfung mit Arzneimitteln wird von vielen Beobachtern als ein Rückschritt in der Kodifizierung der medizinischen Forschung angesehen. Gerade durch die in ihr auszumachende Marginalisierung von Ethik-Kommissionen wird ein gewichtiges prozedurales Prinzip geschwächt. Der vorliegende Band möchte aus interdisziplinärer Perspektive zum Diskurs über die Entstehungsgeschichte, die praktischen Auswirkungen sowie die ethischen Herausforderungen der EU-Verordnung beitragen.
Bd. 28, 2016, 178 S., 39,90 €, br., ISBN 978-3-643-13081-5

LIT Verlag Berlin – Münster – Wien – Zürich – London
Auslieferung Deutschland / Österreich / Schweiz: siehe Impressumsseite

Ethik in der Praxis/Practical Ethics
Studien/Studies
hrsg. von Prof. Dr. Hans-Martin Sass (Universität Bochum/Georgetown University Washington)
Schriftleitung: Dr. Arnd T. May

Tatjana Grützmann
Interkulturelle Kompetenz in der klinisch-ethischen Praxis
Kultursensible Ansätze zum Umgang mit interkulturellen Situationen in der Klinischen Ethikberatung
Aufgrund von Migrationsprozessen, individuellen Lebenskonzepten und multikulturellen Behandlungsteams erleben Mitarbeiter im Gesundheitswesen eine zunehmende kulturelle Diversität und damit verbunden interkulturelle Konfliktsituationen. Anhand von Fallbeispielen werden Lösungswege aufgezeigt und praxisorientierte Techniken zum professionellen Umgang mit derartigen Situationen im klinisch-ethischen Kontext vermittelt. Ansätze für eine kultursensible Ethikberatung, strukturelle Maßnahmen sowie Interkulturelle Kompetenz für Klinikmitarbeiter werden thematisiert und Experten im Rahmen von Interviews hierzu befragt.
Bd. 41, 2016, 244 S., 34,90 €, br., ISBN 978-3-643-13489-9

Hans-Martin Sass
Cultures in Bioethics
Biotopes and Bioethics are highly complex and adaptable systems of Bios. Individual bios is terminal, but the stream of Bios goes on. Basic properties of Bios such as communication and cooperation, competence and competition, contemplation and calculation, compassion and cultivation come in different shades of light and dark in individuals and species, in history and ecology. Hans-Martin Sass discusses the territories of Bios and Bioethics, based on his involvement in decades of consulting in academia, business and politics. Special attention is given to the vision and role of Bioethics in research and training, in religious and cultural traditions, and in the survival, happiness, and health of corporate, social and political bodies.
vol. 40, 2016, 260 pp., 39,90 €, pb., ISBN 978-3-643-90755-4

Simone Horstmann
Ethik der Normalität
Zur Evolution moralischer Semantik in der Moderne
Kann es das *Normale* in der Ethik geben, muss *Normalität* auch dort Berücksichtigung finden, wo mithin einzig Normen regulativen Charakter beanspruchen? Die Arbeit fragt danach, inwieweit Normalität als moralfähige Semantik der Moderne zu verstehen ist. Dabei wird deutlich: Normalität ist der Ethik nicht fremd, sie findet sich vielfach in ethischen Anwendungsdiskursen und kann insbesondere für die Theologische Ethik als moderne Verfeinerung der Natur(rechts)-Semantik aufgefasst werden, die von natural-gegebenen Zweckstrukturen absieht und Moral als Konstruktionsleistung entwirft.
Bd. 39, 2016, 268 S., 34,90 €, br., ISBN 978-3-643-13146-1

Amir Muzur; Hans-Martin Sass (Eds.)
Fritz Jahr and the Foundations of Global Bioethics
The Future of Integrative Bioethics
vol. 37, 2012, 400 pp., 49,90 €, hc., ISBN 978-3-643-90112-5

Ralf Jox; Katja Kühlmeyer; Georg Marckmann; Eric Racine (Eds.)
Vegetative State – A Paradigmatic Problem of Modern Society
Ethical, legal, social and medical perspectives on chronic disorders of consciousness
vol. 36, 2012, 216 pp., 34,90 €, pb., ISBN 978-3-643-90097-5

LIT Verlag Berlin – Münster – Wien – Zürich – London
Auslieferung Deutschland / Österreich / Schweiz: siehe Impressumsseite

Recht der Lebenswissenschaften/Life Sciences and Law
hrsg. von Prof. Dr. Dr. Tade Matthias Spranger (Institut für Wissenschaft und Ethik, Bonn), Prof. Dr. Hans-Georg Dederer (Universität Passau), Prof. Dr. Matthias Herdegen (Universität Bonn), Prof. Dr. Ralf Müller-Terpitz (Universität Mannheim)

Hans-Georg Dederer; Matthias Herdegen
Anbauverbote für gentechnisch veränderte Organismen („Opt-Out")
Nationale Gestaltungsspielräume nach EU-Recht, Welthandelsrecht und Verfassungsrecht
Nach einem fast fünfjährigen Gesetzgebungsverfahren erlaubt das EU-Recht nunmehr den Mitgliedstaaten, den Anbau gentechnisch veränderter Organismen (GVO) zu beschränken oder zu verbieten. Die mit diesem Band vorgelegten Abhandlungen untersuchen die den Mitgliedstaaten eröffneten Gestaltungsspielräume für nationale „Opt-Out"-Maßnahmen. Dabei werden mitgliedstaatlichen Beschränkungen oder Verboten des GVO-Anbaus durch das primäre Unionsrecht sowie das Welthandelsrecht und das Verfassungsrecht enge Grenzen gezogen.
Bd. 10, 2015, 278 S., 29,90 €, br., ISBN 978-3-643-13118-8

Lena H. Laimböck
Totipotenz
Kritik eines normativen Kriteriums im Lichte neuer entwicklungsbiologischer Erkenntnisse
Totipotenz bezeichnet die Fähigkeit zur Ganzheitsbildung. Im Recht wird das naturwissenschaftliche Merkmal herangezogen, um den Embryo zu definieren.
Anlass zur Hinterfragung des Totipotenzkriteriums bieten insbesondere zwei Szenarien: die Erzeugung einer „transienten Totipotenz" und der Einbau von „Entwicklungsbremsen".
Aufbauend auf einer kritischen Analyse des Totipotenzkriteriums entwickelt Lena H. Laimböck als Alternative zu diesem Kriterium das Merkmal der „qualifizierten Entwicklungsfähigkeit" und einen darauf basierenden Reformvorschlag für die einfachrechtliche Embryodefinition.
Bd. 9, 2015, 302 S., 34,90 €, br., ISBN 978-3-643-12967-3

Kurt Fleischhauer
Die Regulierung der medizinischen Versorgung in Deutschland
Normsetzung und Normen in der gesetzlichen und in der privaten Krankenversicherung – Eine Einführung
Die medizinische Versorgung in der gesetzlichen und in der privaten Krankenversicherung wird in Deutschland durch eine Vielzahl von gesetzlichen und untergesetzlichen Normen reguliert. Der Autor beschreibt zunächst den gesetzlichen Rahmen, stellt sodann die an der untergesetzlichen Normsetzung beteiligten Akteure vor und befasst sich anschließend in den zentralen Kapiteln mit den verschiedenen Verfahren der untergesetzlichen Normsetzung und dem wesentlichen Inhalt der Normen. In der Diskussion wird auf die gerichtliche Kontrolle von Normsetzung und Normen eingegangen.
Bd. 8, 2. Aufl. 2015, 248 S., 34,90 €, br., ISBN 978-3-643-12572-9

Isabelle Ruf
Enhancements
Verfassungsrechtliche Aspekte nicht indizierter medizinischer Eingriffe zu Optimierungszwecken
Bd. 7, 2014, 400 S., 44,90 €, br., ISBN 978-3-643-12466-1

Johanna Scherrer
Das Gendiagnostikgesetz
Eine Darstellung unter besonderer Berücksichtigung verfassungsrechtlicher Fragestellungen
Bd. 6, 2012, 512 S., 49,90 €, br., ISBN 978-3-643-11571-3

Anne Fröhlich
Die Kommerzialisierung von menschlichem Gewebe
Eine Untersuchung des Gewebegesetzes und der verfassungs- und europarechtlichen Rahmenbedingungen
Bd. 5, 2012, 464 S., 39,90 €, br., ISBN 978-3-643-11521-8

LIT Verlag Berlin – Münster – Wien – Zürich – London
Auslieferung Deutschland / Österreich / Schweiz: siehe Impressumsseite